P. N. Singer
Time for the Ancients

CHRONOI
Zeit, Zeitempfinden, Zeitordnungen
Time, Time Awareness, Time Management

—

Herausgegeben von

Eva Cancik-Kirschbaum, Christoph Markschies
und Hermann Parzinger

Im Auftrag des Einstein Center Chronoi

Band 3

P. N. Singer
Time for the Ancients

Measurement, Theory, Experience

DE GRUYTER

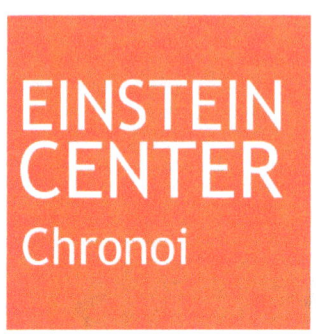

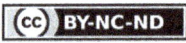

This work is licensed under the Creative Commons Attribution-NonCommercial-NoDerivatives 4.0 International License. For details go to http://creativecommons.org/licenses/by-nc-nd/4.0/.

ISBN 978-3-11-075192-5
e-ISBN (PDF) 978-3-11-075239-7
e-ISBN (EPUB) 978-3-11-075249-6
ISSN 2701-1453

Library of Congress Control Number: 2021948835

Bibliographic information published by the Deutsche Nationalbibliothek
The Deutsche Nationalbibliothek lists this publication in the Deutsche Nationalbibliografie; detailed bibliographic data are available on the Internet at http://dnb.dnb.de.

© 2022 P. N. Singer, published by Walter de Gruyter GmbH, Berlin/Boston
Printing and binding: CPI books GmbH, Leck
www.degruyter.com

Acknowledgements

Institutionally, my gratitude goes to the Wellcome Foundation, which from 2016 to 2019 funded my research project, 'Galen on the Pulse' (grant number 200315/Z/15/Z), from which the present book has partially arisen, and to the Einstein Center Chronoi, Berlin, which supported my further time-related research in the course of two fellowships held between 2019 and 2021, the first physically, the second – during which the book was conceived and completed – virtually. I am also grateful to Birkbeck, University of London, at which the Wellcome grant was held, and to many supportive colleagues there. My thanks go to the whole Chronoi team, as well as to the fellows, who have offered valuable perspectives from a range of scholarly backgrounds, but especially to Stefanie Rabe, Eva Rosentock and Irene Sibbing-Plantholt, for grant- and book-related advice and guidance, and above all for the initial suggestion to write the book. I owe a particular debt of gratitude to Philip van der Eijk, both for initiating my contact with Chronoi and sponsoring my first fellowship there and, much more broadly, for his support of my academic research, first at Newcastle and then in Berlin, since 2009.

I have learnt a huge amount from many colleagues, in London, Berlin and elsewhere. Particularly important for the development of the book, and of my understanding in relevant areas, were my co-fellows during the first Chronoi fellowship: Glen Cooper, Sean Coughlin, Orly Lewis and Christine Salazar. I am grateful to Glen for discussions in Berlin of a number of thorny individual matters related to Galen's *Crises* and *Critical Days*, as well as personal communications by e-mail subsequently. It is difficult to describe my debt to Sean and Orly, with whom I have worked closely for many hours, days and weeks in a collaborative approach to the translation of Galen's works on the pulse (which form a significant part of the textual material for this volume), as well as on many other related areas; my thanks go to them for much that I have learnt on points of detail, as well as for their patience, dedication and support.

Sincere thanks also go to my co-participants in another reading group, David Leith, Ralph Rosen and John Wilkins, who helped refine my understanding and save me from errors in translation of Galen's *Health* (portions of which surface in this volume) – as well as to Chris Gill and my greatly missed friend Piero Tassinari, who participated in that reading group in a previous instantiation.

I am hugely grateful to Catharine Edwards, both for her support during my time at Birkbeck and for a number of individual items of bibliographical and other information.

On completion of a first draft of this book I discovered that Kassandra Miller had also completed a manuscript, *Doctors on the Clock*, which engages with many of the same texts and some of the same issues as the present book, albeit with a different central focus and from a number of different perspectives. I am enormously grateful to Kassandra for her generosity, both in reading and commenting on my draft manuscript and in making a pre-publication draft of hers available to me. I learnt a great deal from both her book and her comments, and the present volume is substantially improved as a result.

I should here also acknowledge that – in keeping with the purpose of the book, as well as the aims of the Chronoi series as a whole, which is partially to present ongoing research in summarized form, not just to publish 'new' material – the section on Galen's account of the different human life stages, in chapter 2, is based closely on the account I give of this in the introduction to my annotated translation of Galen's writings on health in the Cambridge Galen Translation series. Some passages of that translation are also excerpted here, in chapter 1.

Of course, I accumulated many intellectual debts in the time before the immediate period of this research project, not all of which can be itemized here. I must, at least, mention Geoffrey Lloyd, who first stimulated my interest in ancient science, as well as shaping my understanding of it; Tamsyn Barton, who refused to allow me entirely to give it up; and my parents, who – apart from so much else – encouraged my first philosophical speculations, my scientific interests and (perhaps not entirely without justified reservation) my classical studies.

Preface

This book explores ancient Graeco-Roman attitudes to time, its perception, measurement and daily management, and does so with a particular focus on medical approaches and medical sources.

I aim to address such questions as: How did people in the Graeco-Roman world divide organize or divide their days? How did they understand the aging process, or the successive phases of their lives? What was the significance of the changes in the seasons to their daily regimes? What was the relevance of these and other 'cycles' to the understanding of health and disease? What was the role of measurement, and of various technologies of measurement, in these contexts? How did they conceive of their own lives within a broader time span, in relation to – real or imagined – previous ages?

There has been much recent work on time in the ancient world, which has focussed on a number of different topics, especially: calendars and techniques of time measurement; socio-cultural constructions of the lived day, and of different ages or stages of life; attitudes to the past; philosophical speculations, definitions and analyses.[1] But these areas of study have remained to a large extent separate; there is no introductory study offering an overview taking account of them all.

This book aims to fill that gap. At the same time, and while exploring the above questions and offering a synoptic account on the basis of a wide range of sources, it has a particular focus medical writing, and an even more particular one on the work of Galen.

Let me offer a few words by way of explanation of the rationale, first for the focus on medical sources, and secondly for the especial focus on Galen.

Medical writing and medical conceptions constitute a major source of evidence for ancient approaches to and experiences of time, as well as its division and measurement, and the context of this evidence is one of major salience for everyday lives. Medical texts pay closer attention to time than any other literary

---

[1] On time measurement and calendars, as well as on the social and political significance of the latter, see for example: Rüpke (1995), (2011); Schaldach (2001); Hannah (2005), (2008), (2009), (2020); Lehoux (2007); Wolkenhauer (2011); Winter (2013); Bonnin (2015); Graßhoff et al. (2015); Ben-Dov and Doering (2017); Talbert (2017); Bultrighini (2018), (2021a), (2021b); Jones (2020); on daily lives: Ker (2020); Wolkenhauer (2020); on stages of life: Wiedemann (1989); Kleijwegt (1991); Parkin (1999); Laurence (2000); Harlow and Laurence (2002); Scheidel (2001); Cokayne (2003); on attitudes to the past: Csapo and Miller (1998); Darbo-Peschanski (2000); Falkner (1990); Goldhill (2001); de Jong and Nünlist (2007); Richter and Johnson (2017); on philosophical theories: Sorabji (1983) and, on Aristotle, Coope (2005).

sources, on at least three temporal levels: that of precise times within the day (in the context of both health prescriptions and diagnostic observation); that of the seasons of the year (in the context of their relative impact upon health); and that of the human life cycle, from infancy to old age, understood in biological terms. They are thus a very rich – but also a comparatively neglected – source for both theoretical speculation and technological innovation regarding time, and for its experience and management in the ancient world. Amongst other things, they help us to chronicle the growing importance of numbered hours in the Graeco-Roman world and, relatedly, the possible relevance of the growing use of time-telling technologies for everyday time management. A clearer understanding of these developments must at least provide some corrective to the historiographical view which still enjoys considerable currency, that precise time measurement only became important in the conditioning and structuring of everyday lives from the early modern period – still more so to the view that it only achieved real social significance as a function of the modern industrialized workplace.[2]

Moreover, medical texts relating to time offer a distinctive perspective not found in other texts. This is partly a function of the highly contingent, personalized, observation-based, even anecdotal nature of much of the material, which vividly highlights – for example – aspects of individual exercise regimes, diets, sleep patterns and recurrent ailments; details of the daily care of infants or children; or individual experiences and perceptions of the aging process. But the perspective is distinctive in another way too. The medical discourse in some respects offers an alternative model, even a counterblast, to those discourses or traditions which privilege a sacred, social or political calendar. The ambition of medical theory and practice, by contrast, is tendentially to abolish all artificial (or god-given) distinctions between periods of time, acknowledging only those with a biological, environmental or cosmic basis. Thus, while much important recent scholarly work has focused on the calendar, and on the notion of 'festive time', medical perspectives may provide a corrective, or at least a countervailing set of views and experiences. Against a history which tends to privilege tradition and ritual practice, medical sources suggest a view of human experience and human behaviour where differences from one hour, day or month to the next are understood in terms purely of seasonal and biological changes, of environment, diet and daily activity.

---

[2] The point is made strongly by Miller (forthcoming), who mentions as classic statements of such views Thompson (1967); Landes (1983); and, in a similar vein Jenzen and Glasemann (1989); Dohrn-van Rossum (1996).

The rationale for the focus on the second-century-CE doctor and philosopher Galen is partly covered by the above considerations; but it is also the case that his writings happen to include a range of discussions which, taken together, in themselves offer a significant overview of ancient attitudes to time, both within and beyond the medical context. Let me give a brief account of four examples of the unique value of the Galenic material. First, Galen gives the fullest account extant in a literary source of the construction of a sundial, and also of the relationship between sundials and water-clocks. Secondly, he offers by far the richest material for ancient conceptions of different ages, or times of life, and their medical and lifestyle implications. Thirdly, he gives by far the fullest account in our sources of the nature of diagnostic and clinical practice, and how this relates to close temporal observation. Fourthly – and in a more theoretical vein – he presents an original account of our perception of time in relation to motion, and relatedly also of speed and rhythm, which both draws both on existing philosophical accounts and theoretical conceptions and on his clinical experience. This latter discussion – in conjunction with evidence from other medical sources – illuminates ancient views of the extent and limitations of human perception, of the role of quantification, and of rhythm, in both clinical and everyday contexts.

The choice of texts, and the main temporal focus on the second century CE, are partly determined also by considerations of the nature and interrelationship of our surviving sources; and these considerations should be mentioned here too, as they may help to explain what may otherwise seem an unbalanced or eccentric chronological approach. The overwhelming majority of medical sources from the Graeco-Roman world belongs to one of two groups: the so-called 'Hippocratic corpus' on the one hand and the (far more voluminous) works of Galen on the other. The former texts, though spanning a range of dates and authors, were mainly written somewhere in the Greek-speaking world in the fourth or late fifth century BCE,[3] the latter mainly in the second half of the second century CE at Rome. There is a gap of several centuries between these two textual islands, from which period we have very few independently surviving texts, often themselves of uncertain date. Moreover, much of what we *do* know of the medical authors or developments between these two periods – for example, of the important Hellenistic doctors Herophilus and Erasistratus – is from the testimony either of Galen or of authors of even later periods. Galen thus looms very large in our ancient medical evidence, both as an author in his own right and as a source for earlier developments. Moreover (as we shall see especially

---

3 On the problems of the 'Hippocratic corpus' see below, p. 36 with n. 3.

in chapter 3), his works have a close theoretical and ideological relationship with those of the earlier periods, with certain of the 'Hippocratic' works in particular.

For all these reasons, it is difficult to tell anything like a diachronic story of developments in any area related to medical history. I have chosen rather – partly because of this consideration and partly as a function of my own research interests, which have focussed more closely on Galen – to paint a synchronic picture, based mainly in second-century Rome, but at the same time to contextualize this picture with the help of various other texts, some from much earlier periods, but all informing the same intellectual and experiential tradition. In the process, there is inevitably some jumping backwards and forwards, for example between Galen and 'Hippocrates', but it is hoped that such leaps are informative and enriching of that central synchronic picture.

The book thus offers at once a synoptic view of the current state of knowledge of Graeco-Roman thought and practice, in such areas as time measurement and management, approaches to aging, and the perception of time in relation to motion, and also the results of my own and others' latest researches in the specific field of ancient medicine, for example in relation to disease diagnosis or to health prescriptions, which substantially enrich our understanding of these questions.

I should mention a few areas that I do not attempt to address, even synoptically. I give no account here of the relationship of festive to everyday time, or of the extent to which the festive calendar conditioned perceptions of or management of time. The role of both political and religious calendars, and the dedicating of days within the calendar to specific purposes (festive, commercial, juridical, etc.), as well as the related development of a division into either seven-day weeks or eight-day *nundinae*, constitutes a hugely important aspect of the ancient experience and management of time, which has received a comparatively high level of attention in recent literature.[4] These areas have been beyond my scope; moreover, as already suggested, the medical discourse in some ways offers a countervailing historiographical perspective.

Nor, while examining a number of other crucial cycles, do I consider conceptions of cycles of years, arising in either a religious or a philosophical context.[5] Such consideration of the measurement of longer periods of time would poten-

---

4 See especially Hannah (2005), chapters 3 and 5; Rüpke (1995); for further perspectives Beard (1987) and, on the development of the weekly time division in Roman imperial and later times, Bultrighini (2018), (2021a), (2021b).

5 On the ancient Jewish concept of the Sabbatical year, for example, see Carmichael (1999); Casperson (2003); and, for later ramifications, Krinis (2016). Cyclical philosophical notions, meanwhile, would prominently include the Stoic theory of the periodic conflagration of the universe.

tially lead also to analysis of the complex history of the development of the solar calendar and its division into months, and relatedly of the relationship of solar and lunar calendars – again questions not addressed here.[6]

There is much recent work, both within classical studies and within social anthropology, which approaches the question of attitudes to and experience of time from a range of anthropologically-informed theoretical perspectives.[7] The present study does not aim to engage with such theoretical approaches head-on, let alone to advance a new theoretical framework of its own; it does, however, seek to take account of discussions arising in such work where they seem of particular relevance to the specific topics under investigation.

The book is structured in five chapters, each of which takes one large thematic area and aims to consider it from both a broader textual or social perspective and in relation to a more narrowly medical (or in some cases Galenic) perspective. In the first chapter I consider the 'horological scene' of imperial Rome, the importance and the varieties of time measurement and management in daily life, and in particular the division into hours, on the basis of a wide range of sources. This broadly-based account is then followed by a more detailed investigation of the Galenic evidence, both for daily health prescriptions and for the role (and interrelationship) of sundials and water-clocks. In the second chapter, I consider two closely related 'cycles', that of the human lifespan and that of seasons, and the ways that these were conceptualized, experienced or negotiated, both in Graeco-Roman societies more generally and in the medical – especially Hippocratic and Galenic – discourse in particular. Thirdly, and with a main focus on Galen, I consider the two related questions of the (self-)perception or construction of a life or personal biography in the ancient intellectual world and of the attitude to, and nascent periodization of, the past. The fourth chapter investigates the importance of both day and time divisions in ancient diagnostic and clinical practice; it focuses on the crucial medical concepts of *krisis* and *kairos*, also attempting to place these in a broader intellectual and literary context. Finally, I examine Galen's theoretical-philosophical contribution to the discussion of time, both placing this in the broader Greek philosophical tradition and considering its relevance to important clinical and practical questions, in

---

6 See again Hannah (2005), chapter 3, for an intricate account of Greek solutions to the problem, how to divide the year into a regular number of regular months, and of the related question of calculation of dates for periodic festivals such as the Olympics; ibid., chapter 5 for similar issues in Roman calendar-making.
7 Prominent contributions in the former category include van Groningen (1953); de Romilly (1968); Loraux (1986); Bettini (1991); Csapo and Miller (1998); Darbo-Peschanksi (2000); Rosen (2004); in the latter, Good (1968); Gell (1992); Turetzky (1998).

particular the nature of our assessment of time, speed or motion, and the role of qualitative and quantitative elements in this.

As a function of this particular thematic approach, my focus in the book is neither entirely on 'long' nor on 'short' time, to use the terminology adopted in recent literature.[8] While most of the present study is related to a variety of 'short' time units – from hour divisions down to the microscopic divisions theoretically involved in the measurement of the speed of the pulse – I also explore the measurement and conception of time in two 'longer' contexts, that of the ages or phases of life, and that of attitudes to and self-positioning in relation to the past. Moreover, the thematic organization just outlined entails that I do not move neatly either from shorter to longer time units or vice versa, as the various units arise in different ways in relation to the themes successively addressed.

Through its particular focus, the book aims to open a window into some of the most significant questions regarding the ancient awareness, measurement, management, perception and conceptualization of time, and the salience of these to both medical theory and practice and everyday experience.

---

8 See especially the essential work of Miller and Symons (2020).

Contents

List of Illustrations —— XV

List of Tables —— XVII

Chapter One: Time measurement, time management: days, hours and routines —— 1
    Introductory: modes of time measurement at Rome —— 1
    Meridian lines and sundials; seasonal hours —— 4
    Hōrai (ὧραι): from seasons to hours —— 6
    Sundials in the Graeco-Roman world —— 8
    Water-clocks —— 13
    Accuracy —— 17
    Time perception, time management and the use of time-telling devices —— 24
    Medical texts and practices concerning time management —— 27
    Galen against 'festive time' —— 33

Chapter Two: Times of life and times of year: the ever-shifting cycles —— 35
    Introductory —— 35
    The cycle of life: the ages of man (and woman) in the Graeco-Roman world —— 36
    Medical authors on the life stages —— 43
    The yearly cycle: the seasons —— 51
    Non-periodic disease recurrence: some endless cycles —— 61
    Conclusion regarding medical discussions of cycles —— 63
    A final consideration: temporal and atemporal human beings —— 64

Chapter Three: Lives in time: history, biography, bibliography —— 67
    The old and the new —— 72
    Galen on the old and the new (1): the ideology of the ancient —— 74
    Galen on the old and the new (2): historiography and periodization —— 83
    Galen on his own age —— 89
    Galen on his own life and works —— 91
    A parallel biography: Porphyry's *Life of Plotinus* —— 98

Chapter Four: Time for the doctor: crises, perils and opportunities —— 102
    Kairos, *krisis* and *peira*: a perilous time —— 102

Periodic diseases —— 106
Fevers and their recurrence: Hippocrates; Galen; Galen's rivals —— 108
Non-Galenic views: over-simplification and over-complication —— 109
Galen's own schemes —— 116
Reconciling theory, observation and authority: Galen's medical month —— 117

Chapter Five: Time, motion, rhythm: reality, perception and quantification —— 123
Philosophical questions and the relationship of time to motion —— 124
Galen on time (1): evidence for his theoretical analysis —— 128
Galen on time (2): further analysis and justification —— 132
Galen on speed: the measurement of the pulse —— 136
Minimal units of time (1): the atomic nature of time perception —— 148
Minimal units of time (2): the analysis of rhythm —— 152
Summary on minimal time units in Aristoxenus, Herophilus and Galen —— 158
An isolated case of quantification? Pulse rate and the water-clock —— 159
Conclusion —— 162

Bibliography —— 165
Primary Texts —— 165
Citation conventions and abbreviations —— 165
List of primary sources cited —— 166
Secondary Literature —— 170

Index of names —— 181

General index —— 184

List of Illustrations

Figure 1   The *horologium Augusti* as depicted on the base of the Column of Antoninus Pius in Rome
Figure 2   The three great Augustan monuments – mausoleum, Ara Pacis and *horologium* – in the northern Campus Martius in Rome
Figure 3   Some examples of sundials in the Graeco-Roman world
Figure 4   An Egyptian outflow water-clock
Figure 5   Ctesibius' sophisticated water-clock
Figure 6   Diagram of Galen's account of the design of a water-clock
Figure 7   The two-sphere model of the cosmos, with the zodiac and planets
Figure 8   The heliacal rising of the Pleiades, Hyades and Orion
Figure 9   'Mundus homo annus': the mediaeval circle of correspondences of elements, seasons, fluids and ages
Figure 10 A Roman funerary inscription recording a lifespan in years, months, days and hours
Figure 11 *Kairos* personified as a dashing youth, with a knife and scales
Figure 12 The bedside as battlefield: Galen correctly diagnosing the illness of the emperor Marcus Aurelius, surrounded by rival physicians.
Figure 13 Calculating the period (wrongly): Galen's conversion table in *Periods*
Figure 14 The fine-tuning of the senses (1): tuning a lyre
Figure 15 The fine-tuning of the senses (2): the hands and the pulse

List of Tables

Table 1 Ages in the 'Hippocratic' *Hebdomads*
Table 2 A standard 'Hippocratic' age division (from *Regimen* 1.33)
Table 3 The stages of life in Galen
Table 4 Divisions of the seasons (according to *Regimen*)
Table 5 Galen's typology of fevers
Table 6 The mediaeval circle of correspondences: 'world – man – year'
Table 7 Galen's periodization of the past

Chapter One:
Time measurement, time management: days, hours and routines

In this chapter I explore Graeco-Roman techniques of, and attitudes towards, time measurement, from the twin perspectives of everyday life and medicine. I survey literary and archaeological evidence for the two main available technologies of time measurement, sundials and water-clocks, and consider what this evidence tells us about their differential accessibility and context of use, and about Roman attitudes to daily or hourly time organization. I then proceed to examine further some literary, and, in more detail, some medical texts which shed light on ancient attitudes to time management and the division of the day; on the importance of, and relationship between, the two forms of time measurement, as well as the relationship of seasonal to equinoctial hours; and on the balance of work and leisure, in particular exercise, activities within such daily time divisions.

Introductory: modes of time measurement at Rome

An obelisk towered high over the Campus Martius in Rome. Built in 10/9 BCE, the *horologium* of the emperor Augustus cast its shadow over a long stretch of the low-lying area, where a metal line and markings had been laid in the ground. It was itself visible from a great distance and complemented two other great Augustan edifices in the same area: the Mausoleum Augusti and the Ara Pacis. (See figures 1 and 2.) The line on the ground ran due north from the obelisk: a meridian, which the shadow hit at noon each day. The markings along its length indicated different dates, and these would be hit by the shadow at noon on successive days, as it grew longer or shorter in the course of the year.

Prominently placed above the forum, meanwhile – the centre of both legal and commercial activity in the city – were one or two sundials, visibly dividing the passing time of daylight into twelve equal units, which, by the late second century CE, the date of the texts which we shall focus on in this chapter, had stood there for more than three hundred years. Other, equally publicly visible, sundials were features of cities throughout the Graeco-Roman world.[1]

---

[1] For detail and for an account of the early Roman history of time measurement, and for the historical sequence of publicly accessible markers of time in the city, see Wolkenhauer

OpenAccess. © 2022 Singer, published by De Gruyter. This work is licensed under the Creative Commons Attribution-NonCommercial-NoDerivatives 4.0 International License.
https://doi.org/10.1515/9783110752397-004

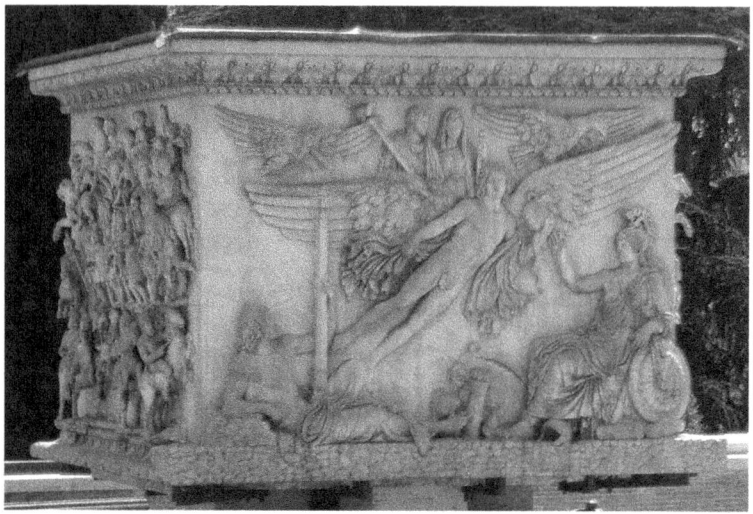

Figure 1: The *horologium Augusti* as depicted on the base of the Column of Antoninus Pius in Rome. An obelisk emerges from the lap of the personified Campus Martius; a winged figure, possibly Eternity (*Aiōn*) conducts Antoninus and Faustina to the heavens. The column base is now in the Vatican Museums. Image: https://commons.wikimedia.org/wiki/File:Musei_vaticani_-_base_colonna_antonina_01106.JPG

A few steps from those public sundials, the ancient visitor to the forum – if by chance business affairs took him into the Basilica Aemilia et Fulvia – would find an equally venerable instrument of time measurement, a water-clock or *clepsydra*, placed there in the year 159 BCE, and dividing the day into (probably) half hours.

Water-clocks, indeed, had the capacity to measure much smaller units of time than that. The main attested use of the *clepsydra* was, as we shall see, in legal contexts; but here the water-clocks in question were simple outflow devices, whose sole function was the demarcation of short, distinct blocks of time. At the other end of the technological spectrum, an elaborate and sophisticated *clepsydra* might constitute a luxury object or perhaps status symbol, for example

---

(2020), esp. 218–20. The main literary source is Pliny, *Natural History* 7.60.212–15. The Twelve Tables made reference only to the moments of sunrise and sunset, which were publicly displayed on the Rostra; the public announcement of noon was a somewhat later innovation; and Pliny records accounts of a first sundial erected either at the Temple of Quirinus, eleven years before the Pyrrhic War (i.e. c. 295 BCE), or at the Rostra during the First Punic War (c. 262 BCE). He adds that this sundial was obeyed for many years although inaccurate, and a new one was erected c. 164 BCE. See also Hannah (2009): 134–6, and further note 12 below.

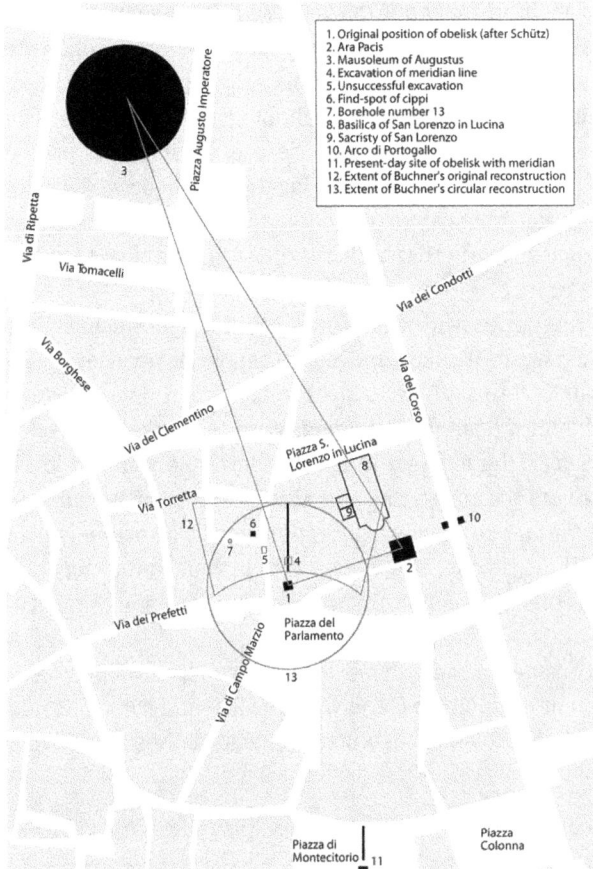

Figure 2: The three great Augustan monuments – mausoleum, Ara Pacis and *horologium* – in the northern Campus Martius in Rome. The plan, showing the monuments in their positions on a map of the modern city, also indicates their ancient prominence and interrelationship. Note that nos. 12 and 13 show the dubious reconstructions of the monument as a sundial, by Buchner, while no. 4 shows its actual function as a meridian line. The image is reproduced by kind permission of Peter Heslin from his article (2007).

in the dining room of a well-to-do citizen, whose guests might pass a little time admiring the ingenuity and luxury of their host's most up-to-date acquisition.[2] Such a water-clock might be capable of measuring hours and even subdivisions

---

[2] Petronius describes a rich man boasting of his water-clock (*Satyricon* 26); cf. Pliny, *Letters* 3.1.8.

of hours, of both day and night, throughout the year, with impressive accuracy. Some water-clocks were also on prominent display, certainly by the second century CE, in a number of public spaces – for example at gymnasia, theatres or sanctuaries – although little is known of their technological specifications or measuring capabilities.³ There is also evidence of the use, again in the private context, of handheld or portable sundials. These again would be objects for the elite, probably not of great practical value and certainly not in widespread use. Archaeological evidence suggests that both handheld sundials and sophisticated water-clocks were a rarity.⁴

These few examples present us with a way into the world of ancient time awareness and time management. We have moved, in this brief overview, from the most publicly accessible forms of time measurement in Rome – which were at the same times the ones dealing in the largest units, marking the position of the day within the year, the moment of midday or, at the smallest level, the division the day into hours – through those used in business and legal contexts, in which it was important to have a conception and a measurement of smaller units, to the level of the private, elite household, in which more accurate devices might have been rather a diversion than something of serious practical value.

We shall proceed to consider in more detail the physical construction, context and use of these different technologies, and what these – and some relevant texts – tell us about ancient attitudes to time management, daily organization, leisure and punctuality.

Meridian lines and sundials; seasonal hours

The spectacularly public monument with which we began functioned both as a calendar, showing the moment of the year that had been reached, and as a daily indicator of noon. The information laid out on the ground for the first of these purposes – the marks along the meridian line's length – included such labels as 'beginning of spring' and 'Etesian winds' (whose arrival early in the summer was a well-known marker of the beginning of the safe sailing season), as well as the names of the zodiac signs and a mark for each degree of the zodiac. On its progress from its shortest extent, at the summer solstice, to its longest, at the winter solstice, the shadow came level with a series of markings on one side

---

3 See further p. 24 with n. 31 below.
4 See Talbert (2017); Jones (2020): 125.

of the line, where letters are to be found mentioning the zodiac signs of the late summer to winter months, as well as others corresponding to specific moments in that half of the year; as the shadow shortened on successive days between December and June, the corresponding markings were to be read on the other side of the line.

The utility of such a meridian line, then, is twofold. Passers-by would be made aware of the approach and passing of midday, although of no smaller division of the day than that; but this in itself may have assisted in the regulation and organization of their day. But the observer of the shadow at midday would also gain a confirmation of the position within the calendar on any given day. One chief aim of the construction may indeed have been to give reassurance of stability, to make an assertion of the new era or reliability of the calendar that was to result from Augustus' taking of control over the calendar after a period of drift and uncertainty. The reliability of the new system, after Augustus' reforms and adjustments, would be manifest from the agreement of the lines visibly marked on the ground with the days and festivals of the civic calendar. Indeed, the purpose of the instrument was at least as much to impress and dominate as it was to inform; there was, as a number of scholars have pointed out, a clear political message to be read, not just in the *horologium*'s visibility from afar, but also in its proximity to and physical relationship with the other two great Augustan monuments in the area, mentioned above.[5]

We might say, then, that the *horologium Augusti* is both misnamed and a somewhat unusual case: not in fact a sundial, not a 'teller of the hours', but

---

5 See especially Heslin (2007) and (2019), emphasizing both the ideological or propaganda function of the meridian – giving visible form to Augustus' reform and stabilization of the calendar, and mutually reinforcing the other two major Augustan monuments in the northern area of the Campus Martius – and its role in 'making Rome run on time'. Augustus had taken control of the calendar on his adoption of the role of *pontifex maximus* on the death of Lepidus the previous year, and had instituted adjustments that had become necessary as a result of an inaccurate intercalation of leap days (three instead of four) in leap years in the time of Julius Caesar, and a failure to address this for more than thirty years. Heslin, following Schütz, rejects the role previously attributed to the *horologium*, especially by Buchner, as a sundial, with a large physical presence on the ground of the Campus Martius. (A further controversial aspect, explored especially by Heslin 2019, is the probable re-laying of the meridian – and appropriation of the ideological message of the monument – by the emperor Domitian, nearly a century later.) While the controversy has continued, a broad consensus now favours the view of the *horologium* as a meridian line and *not* a sundial. Important further discussions of the role and significance of the monument are given by Zanker (1988); Barton (1995); Rehak (2006); Hannah (2011); the controversy, and history of the archaeological excavations, is summarized both by Heslin and by Haselberger (2011), (2014). On the public aspect of calendars more generally see Rüpke (1995), (2011).

rather, as we have seen, a teller of progress through the year, as well as a marker of the crucial time of noon. Yet this calendrical function was an important one. Indeed, it was probably the original function, from Archaic Greek times, of the first kinds of gnomon, from which the more recognizable 'sundial' developed. That is to say, publicly visible gnomons functioned in earlier times as tellers of the seasons (and of midday on each day), not as tellers of hours – and it is possible that this remained an important function of some such constructions even in the imperial period.[6]

On the question of nomenclature: while some scholars now prefer '*solarium*' or 'meridian', I have kept here to the traditional '*horologium*'. The original Greek term, ὡρολόγιον, literally a reckoner or teller of *hōrai*, could, after all, refer to the calculation of *seasons*, not just of *hours*.

Hōrai (ὧραι): from seasons to hours

Now, this terminological decision, while unimportant in itself, leads us on to a point which is by contrast of very considerable importance for the story that we are telling. For behind the semantic range of the Greek term ὥρα (*hōra*) lies a historical development which is crucial to the history of time measurement itself – a development which, though difficult to trace with complete accuracy, took place at some point after the Greek Archaic period.

We should pause to investigate these important developments – both the semantic one and its relative in everyday life – before returning to our survey of the Roman imperial horological *mise-en-scène*.

The Greek word ὥρα (*hōra*), in its earliest occurrences, in Archaic Greek literature, refers not to hours but either to times in a more general sense or, more

---

[6] The earliest Greek gnomon, the invention of which is attributed to Anaximander by Diogenes Laertius (*Lives of the Eminent Philosophers* 2.1; cf. Pliny, *Natural History* 2.78.187), very probably had *only* this function, of tracking the sun's motion through the seasonal year by marking the lengths of the shadow at noon; it is unclear whether Anaximander's technology extended also to the measuring of hours. However, a division into twelve hours at an early period is attested by Herodotus, who attributes its origin to the Babylonians (*Histories* 2.109.3). (Both the sundial technology and the hour division existed earlier in Egypt and Mesopotamia, and arrived in the Greek-speaking world from that source. It is possible, indeed, that the twelve-fold division mentioned by Herodotus was in fact a division of the whole of the day and night, corresponding to the Babylonian division into twelve *beru* or 'double hours'.) On these questions, as well as the archaeological evidence for the early development of the sundial, see Hannah (2009), chapter 4; and on the relationship of sundial and calendar see Hannah (2020). The possible semantic range of the term *horologium* is a point made by Miller (forthcoming).

specifically, to seasons of the year. Nor is there any other word at this period which denotes 'hours', in the sense of certain units into which the day is divided. Even by the fourth century BCE, the use of the word to refer to hours is at best insecurely attested. The point is of particular significance from the medical perspective. Only two passages in the so-called 'Hippocratic corpus' mention the significance of *hōrai* in the course of a disease; of these, one is attributable to a date later than that of the core corpus (late fifth – early fourth century BCE), while the other is textually insecure.[7]

The use of the term *hōra* to refer to an hour, then, is insecurely attested, even as the late as the fourth century; and this semantic situation seems to correspond to a sociological one, whereby – in spite of the advent of a technology capable of dividing the day into equal parts by some time in the fifth century, attested by Herodotus (see n. 6 above) – the hour probably did not come to be widely used as a unit for practical, in particular medical, purposes, until considerably later.

By some time in the third century BCE, on the other hand, the use of seasonal hours seems to have been widespread, including for administrative purposes. Such use is for example attested by papyri, some of which give evidence of the use of hour-markings within a postal system which had become established under the Ptolemies; the first secure medical reference to hours seems also to belong to a similar period.[8]

The development is of considerable significance for the medical assessment and measurement of time, which will be a particular focus in this study. As we shall see later in this chapter in the context of daily regimes for health, and also in chapter 4 in the context of the analysis and diagnosis of diseases of periodic recurrence, the identification of precise hours within the day was of great theo-

---

[7] The two instances are at *Internal Affections* (27, 148 Loeb, VII.238 L.), which is very probably a later text) and *Epidemics* 4, 94 Loeb (V.150 L.), which probably dates to the fourth century, but where the correct reading is almost certainly not τρίτην ὥρην ('third hour') but τὴν αὐτὴν ὥρην 'the same time' (as adopted by Potter in the Loeb): the latter is a common phrase in the *Epidemics*, whereas there is no other such instance of numerical precision. See Langholf (1973); Miller (forthcoming). (More broadly on problems surrounding the dating of, and indeed the very term, 'Hippocratic corpus', see below, p. 36 with n. 3.) The earliest text where the equation ὥρα = hour has been made is otherwise Plato's *Laws* 6, 784a–b. This interpretation, which is far from certain, is advanced by Sattler (2020); her argument at the same time clearly brings out the absence of any such reference to or employment of short time units *before* the date of the *Laws*, including elsewhere in Plato's oeuvre.

[8] For hour markers used in the postal service see Remijsen (2007); the medical reference is the attribution to the New Comic poet Machon of the statement: 'you will die during the seventh hour' (by Athenaeus, *Dinner Sophists* 341a–b).

retical importance for doctors in the imperial period. Moreover, these doctors are, at least in some cases, claiming to base themselves in detail on the prescriptions and theoretical models of the 'classical' texts of the so-called Hippocratic corpus. Yet a very significant development has taken place between the two periods and between the two sets of practitioners. Divisions of the day made in the Hippocratic corpus, in observational or prescriptive contexts, are either approximate or described in terms of bodily events ('the middle of the day', 'on waking', 'after food', etc.), rather than in terms of numbered hours. This contrasts sharply with the divisions of, say, Galen or the Methodists. Similarly, while the analysis of periodically recurring diseases is certainly present in the Hippocratic corpus, and indeed functions as a framework for that offered by the imperial-period practitioners, the Hippocratic calculation (implicit or explicit) is in terms of days, whereas both Galen and his rivals operate complex numerical models according to which the identification of precise numerical hours is of immense diagnostic significance.

We shall consider these conflicting imperial-period models, and their relationship with their Hippocratic forebears, in detail below. For the moment we confine ourselves to noting the transition from a medical world in which the smallest numbered unit of division is the day to one in which twelve hours of the day, and twelve of the night, may all assume diagnostic or prescriptive value, and therefore require – in theory at least – to be accurately measured.[9]

Sundials in the Graeco-Roman world

Let us return then to our survey of the Roman horological scene. From the Hellenistic period onward, sundials were erected in cities throughout the ancient Mediterranean, and had become widespread by the imperial period. They undoubtedly had the function of telling the hours of the day, in an accessible and publicly visible manner.

This was, however, not their only function. Before proceeding to discuss the technology and its dispersion over the empire in more detail, we should reflect on the senses in which the public erection or dedication of sundials may have had a symbolic, as much as a practical, value. (Such reflection will be relevant later in the chapter, too, when we look at the extent to which sundials were or

---

[9] This transition is a major theme of Miller (forthcoming), who argues, relatedly, that precise temporal measurement, using the technologies of sundials and water-clocks, was a central feature of imperial-period medicine.

were not in fact relied upon, in particular by doctors, in the regulation of everyday life.)

A number of considerations point towards such symbolic, and sometimes ornamental, significance. It has been suggested, for example, that the prominent presence of sundials at a number of sanctuaries betokens a ritualistic or semiotic role – that in this context they function as an abstract representation of 'time' or 'eternity', or in some cases make reference to the sun-god. There is, further, some evidence that the erection of sundials in Roman colonies is a function of the desire by local elites to demonstrate their 'Romanness', to adopt or establish Roman temporal norms. Perhaps most significantly, the presence of sundials in certain kinds of portrait image makes clear their iconographical value as symbolic of *paideia* – of the Greek model of education and philosophical knowledge, and in particular of an assertion by Romans of their adoption of it, of the status of the person in question as *pepaideumenos*, cultured or educated in this Greek sense. In such images, a man is depicted with beard and cloak – other standard images of philosophy or *paideia* – and alongside a sundial or sphere representing the cosmos. The euergetic dedication of a sundial, alongside that of a sphere, might also have such symbolic, as well as religious or theological, significance. Moreover, the highly elaborate, but not easily readable, design of at least *some* sundials, suggests their function as a visible celebration of ingenuity, rather than a pragmatic artefact. It is possible to argue – conversely – that the inaccuracy and poor workmanship of many extant sundials, especially those found at Pompeii, also suggest a symbolic or ornamental, rather than a practical, value.[10]

Let us consider the technology of the sundials themselves in a little more detail. Roman sundials divided the entire span of daylight time on each day into twelve equal hours. That is to say, they measured the *seasonal* hours, which vary in length throughout the year, not the hours of equal length (*equinoctial* hours) familiar to us in modern time-keeping. (The technology and calculations enabling a sundial to perform the latter task were an innovation of a later period,

---

10 See Hannah (2020: 336), suggesting that sundials at sanctuaries of Apollo 'reflect an actualization ... of the identification of Apollo with Helios the Sun-God'. On portrait images of a *pepaideumenos* with sphere and/or sundial see Marrou (1938); Ewald (1999); Lang (2012): 80–109, and cf. Borg (2004a); Bonnin (2013). On the broader notions of *paideia* and *pepaideumenos* in Roman imperial culture see Borg (2004b); Richter and Johnson (2017). It is worth noting here – and in relation to Galen's reflections on sundials, which we shall consider later in the chapter – that such a dedication of a cosmic sphere at Pergamum, accompanied by a poem celebrating both the heavenly and the geometrical bodies, is very probably due to Galen's father; cf. Singer (2019a). The decorative rather than practical value of some sundials, especially in later Roman times, is discussed by Miller (forthcoming).

first evidenced in the mediaeval Islamicate world.) Roman sundials were constructed on a number of different models: some have a planar construction, laid out either horizontally or vertically; there are convex and conical, alongside concave, designs; some consist of two parts for two sets of hours. (See figure 3.)

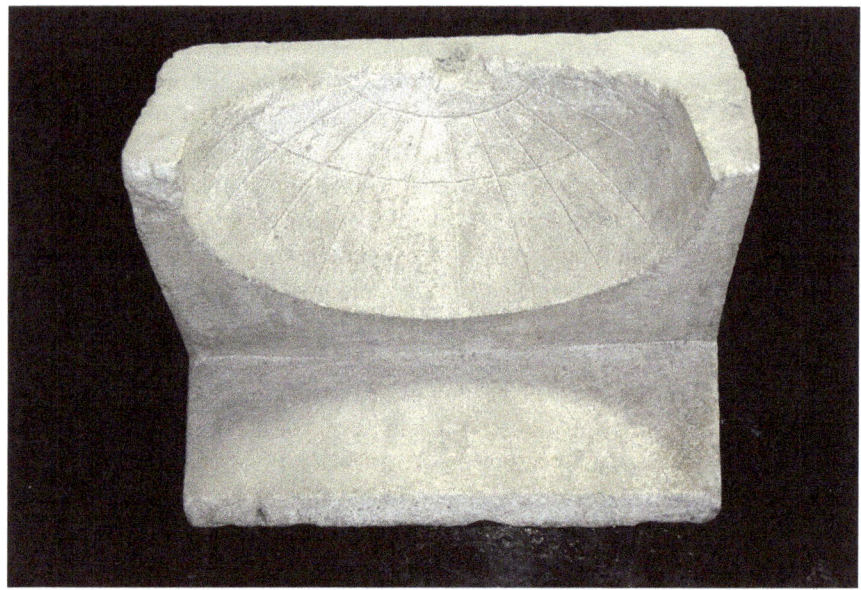

Figure 3a: Concave sundial, Rome, unknown date, held by Museo Nazionale Romano, image from: Berlin Sundial Collaboration, Image of Dialface ID 35, Rome Inventory Nr. 540244, 2015, Ancient Sundials, Edition Topoi, DOI: 10.17171/1-1-5798

Overwhelmingly the most common design, however, is that in which a vertical gnomon casts its shadow onto lines inscribed in a concave section of a sphere. Here, too, we should consider the object's symbolic or didactic significance: as Jones has suggested, we should see such a sundial not just as a time-telling instrument but also as a 'didactic image of the foundations of geometrical astronomy'.[11] That is to say, such concave sundial constructions may be taken as partial representations of the celestial sphere – the sphere, that is, to which the stars are attached, and which surrounds and rotates about the earth.[12]

Whichever the precise design, however, the fundamental principle is the same. The shadow of the sun, cast by the gnomon, will reach eleven different

---

[11] Jones (2016): 25.
[12] For this 'two-sphere' model of the cosmos see below, p. 52–4, with figure 7.

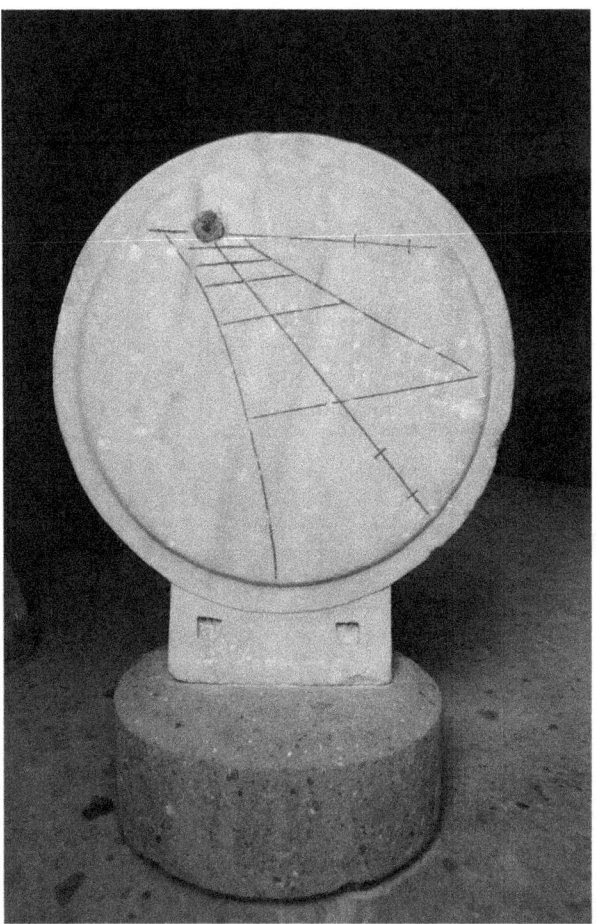

Figure 3b: Vertical planar sundial, image from: Berlin Sundial Collaboration, Ancient Sundials, Dialface ID 276, Grottaferrata, Inv. Nr. 1217, 2014, Edition Topoi, DOI: 10.17171/1-1-2973

marker lines in the course of the sun's perceived progress through the sky, hitting a different point on that line according to its varying height through the year. The sundials almost invariably have eleven such lines (though occasionally the division is into some other number than twelve, e.g. fourteen). Further subdivision, for example into half hours, was not done (although within at least some of the models it would have been in principle quite possible). There is then, typically, a further set of lines, crossing the hour lines, and corresponding to the different length of the shadows at different times of the year; the combination of the

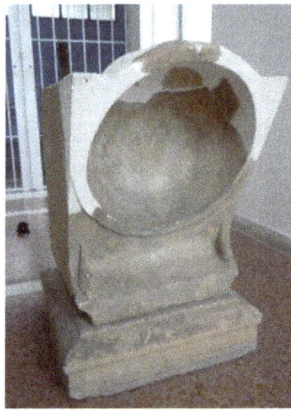

Figure 3c: Roofed spherical sundial, from Tinos, first century BCE, image from: Berlin Sundial Collaboration, Ancient Sundials, Dialface ID 283, Tinos, Inv. Nr. A139, 2014, Edition Topoi, DOI: 10.17171/1-1-3077

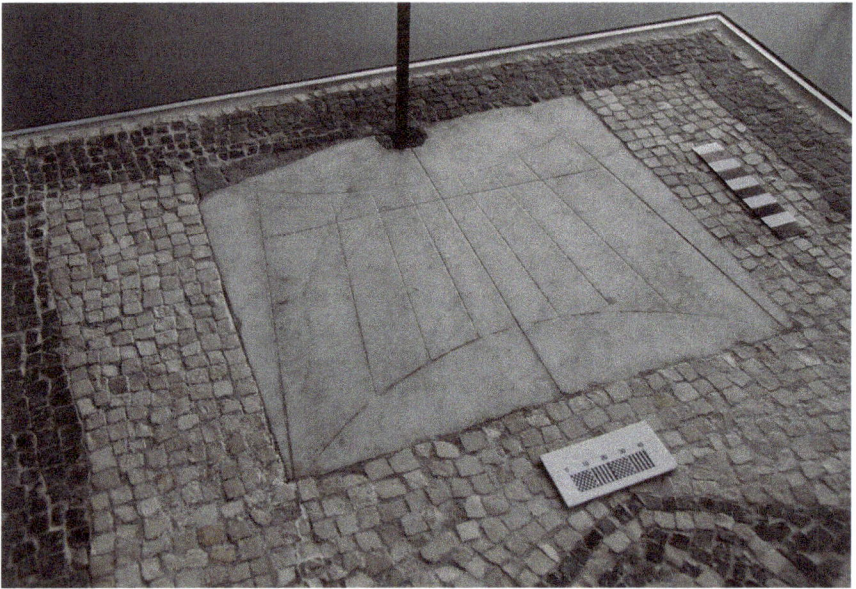

Figure 3d: Horizontal planar sundial, Schaldach, Karlheinz, Image of Dialface ID 629, Frankfurt, 2015, Ancient Sundials, Edition Topoi, DOI: 10.17171/1-1-8421

two sets of lines enables the viewer to read each hour off at the right point at any time of the year.[13]

---

[13] On the historical developments, and the variety of designs of sundial, in the Greek and Roman worlds, see especially Jones (2020): 131–6; further Schaldach (2001); Hannah (2009),

The 'hours' thus measured, then, would be of 60 minutes' duration only at the two equinoxes, and would depart gradually further from that length the further one moved from either of these towards either of the solstices. The maximum discrepancy between the 60-minute hour and the seasonal one, at the latitude of Rome, is 15 minutes in each direction. That is to say, a seasonal hour at the summer solstice lasts 75 minutes, at the winter solstice 45. The Roman system of time-keeping or referring to times of the day, familiar from literary texts and continuing in Europe until mediaeval times, was based on this way of dividing the day. 'At the sixth hour' refers to midday, that is the moment of completion of the sixth hour since dawn or the moment 'of first light' (*prima luce*); 'at the twelfth hour' means sunset; and so on for the other hours between those points. The night was similarly divided into twelve hours, which again varied seasonally; here there was an additional principle of division, arising from the military context: that of the 'watches', each four hours in duration.[14]

The purpose of the sundial, then, though partially symbolic, would also be to regulate time, or assist in time management, for a general public. People would be able to observe the arrival of midday, but also, in more detail, what hour it was at any moment (given enough sunlight, of course), and would be assisted in the making and keeping of appointments – for example, to meet at someone's house 'at the eighth hour' – on a tolerably agreed basis.

Water-clocks

The use of a water-clocks, in a specifically legal or political context, goes back to classical Athenian times. Here the *clepsydra* in question has a simple and single function, namely to measure the passing of a specific segment of time. In the context of the Athenian lawcourt, it was important that speakers were allowed equal amounts of time for their speeches, and that the timespans in question

---

chs 4 and 6; Winter (2013); and also the database of archaeological finds and images of Graßhoff et al. (2015).

14 Pliny the Elder (*Natural History* 33.32.97–8) mentions the measurement of both day and night shifts by lamps, for men engaged in the constant labour of baling water out of Spanish silver mines ('noctibus diebusque ... lucernarum mensura'). By this are presumably meant oil lamps, which, given a certain size, amount of oil, etc., would burn for a known period of time. A similar use of oil lamps to determine time is mentioned in some magical papyri; see Betz (1986): 172–82 and 336; Hannah (2009): 96–7, with n. 3. A form of water-clock is also attested for the measurement of night watches; this is adjustable in volume, to enable it to measure the hours on longer shorter nights: Aeneas Tacticus 22.24–5; Hannah (2009): 108.

were previously agreed, known units. Thus, a perforated vessel of a given size is filled with water, and the time allotted for a speech is the time taken for that vessel to empty, or some multiple of this. The smallest such time unit was provided by the *chous* ('jug', also used as a standard measure of volume, roughly equivalent to a modern litre, or 1.7 pints), which would give a time of somewhere in the region of three to six minutes.[15]

It is important to note that this technology, in this simple form, does not allow further subdivision of the block of time represented by the vessel, since the speed of flow changes in the course of the vessel's emptying. Marks placed at equal vertical intervals on the side of the vessel would not correspond to equal divisions of time. This shortcoming may, of course, be rectified, through a calibration of the sides of the vessel based on careful calculation or observation of the varying speed of the outflow over the whole period. The development of such precisely calibrated outflow clocks does not, however, seem to have taken place to any great extent in the Graeco-Roman world. In Egypt, by contrast, outflow water-clocks were used, both at a much earlier period than is attested for Greece, and with much greater sophistication of design. Here, it seems that the main context of their use was a religious one.[16] (See figure 4.)

The basic classical Greek form of the water-clock, with its original legal context, however, contrasts with a range of more sophisticated inventions, which had been developed in Hellenistic times and were available to the Romans. These more sophisticated water-clocks came in a variety of designs, some with markings on the side of a vessel, some showing the passing of the time with a dial. The crucial innovation here, for which our main source is the Roman archi-

---

15 But there are other versions than this completely straightforward one attested, even for the earlier period; cf. nn. 16 and 17 below. See Wolkenhauer (2020): 227, with further literature; Hannah (2009): 99–102, assembling the texts that mention the *clepsydra* in the fifth- and fourth-century Athenian legal and political context, especially ps.-Aristotle, *Athenian Constitution* 69, Aeschines, *The False Embassy* 126; Demosthenes, *Against Makartatos* 8 (which all mention, or complain of, the various numbers of *choes* allotted for speeches in different contexts); Demosthenes sometimes uses the word 'water' on its own to indicate this form of time measurement, e.g. *Against Euboulides* 21; *Against Konon* 36; *Against Stephanos* 1.8; *On the Crown* 139; cf. Plato, *Theaetetus* 172d. As Hannah also points out (ibid. 101), some form of *clepsydra* is reported to have been in the past also for the timing of plays (Aristotle, *Poetics* 7, 1451a7–9) and even – though perhaps jokingly – for meetings with a prostitute (Athenaeus, *The Dinner Sophists* 13, 567c–d). Further on the technology and its development Winter (2013), and for a summary Hannah (2013a).
16 See von Lieven and Schomberg (2020), esp. 58 on the Egyptian dates (going back to at least the sixteenth century), and 68–9 on questions of calibration and design.

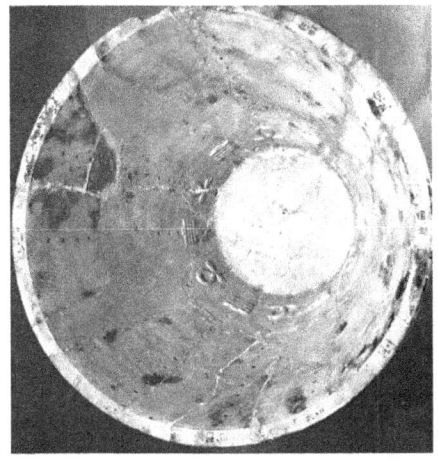

Figure 4: An Egyptian outflow water-clock; on the inside are markers corresponding to the different hours at different months. It is noteworthy that surviving Greek or Roman outflow clocks seldom attain to or attempt such precision, their most common purpose being the delineation of a single block of time which is not further subdivided. Image from Desroches-Noblecourt (1976), 41.

tectural author Vitruvius, is attributed to a Hellenistic-period inventor, Ctesibius.[17]

Here, the fundamental principle of operation – unlike that of the basic water-clocks just described – is that of inflow of water to a vessel at constant speed. A measuring vessel (A) is filled up at constant speed; the essential requirement that enables this is a mechanism whereby the water supplied to vessel A comes from another vessel (B), in which the level of the water is kept always constant. The constant level of water in vessel B ensures constant pressure, which in turn ensures a constant speed of outflow from vessel B, and thus into vessel A. This allows the time represented by the filling of vessel A as a whole to be subdivided, in principle into as small units as one wishes. (See figure 5.)

So, a mechanism of outflow at variable speed has been replaced by one of inflow at constant speed; and this enables further measurable subdivision. Once

---

[17] For the historical developments and the variety of literary and archaeological sources see Lewis (2000); Hannah (2009), ch. 5. A very useful account with helpful illustrations is Landels (1979). Our main literary source for the more sophisticated water-clocks is Vitruvius, who describes in detail the designs of the Hellenistic inventor Ctesibius (*Architecture* 9.8.4–15); he also describes a still more elaborate construction which combines telling the time with a display of the positions of the heavenly bodies, and in particular of the zodiac (*Architecture* 9.8.8–15). Vitruvius even credits Ctesibius with the invention, through the use of the related technology of the water organ, of a water-clock that 'trumpeted' (i.e. an early form of alarm clock), *Architecture* 12.11; cf. Athenaeus, *Dinner Sophists* 4, 174c, claiming that Plato also had some such device at his disposal.

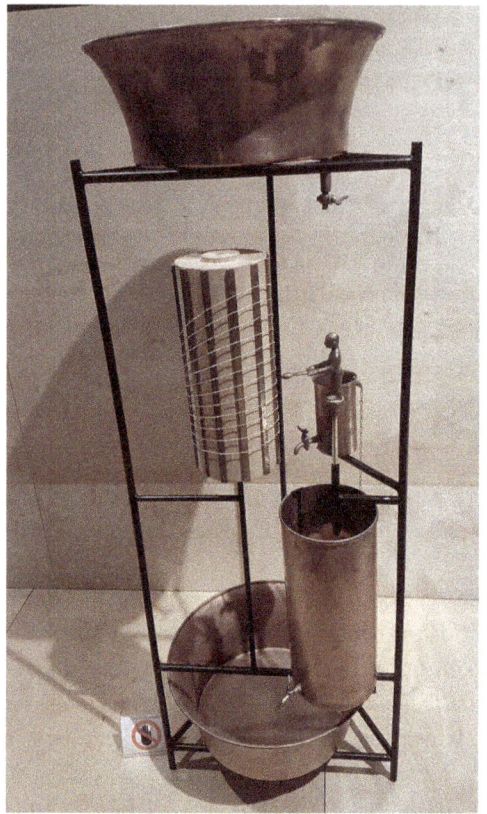

Figure 5: Ctesibius' sophisticated water-clock. There have been many attempts to reconstruct the design of this water-clock, following its description by Vitruvius. This one is from the Archaeological Museum of Thessaloniki. Image source: https://commons.wikimedia.org/wiki/File:Ctesibius%27s_water_clock,_3rd_century_BC,_Alexandria_(reconstruction).jpg

filled, the vessel must be emptied, or the process restarted; or there may have been even more sophisticated mechanisms which performed that process without intervention.

As already suggested, however, the use of such complex and elaborate devices in Roman society was at best confined to elite circles, and probably a rarity even there. The main context of the use of the *clepsydra* – both as a term and as a physical reality – continued to be that of the lawcourt. The intense demands of this technically complex, professionalized and conflictual legal environment required time measurement at a much finer and more precise level than was apparently needed in any other context in Roman society.[18] Thus, for example, the orator Cicero makes a derogatory reference to 'barking against the *clepsydra*', and Pliny the Younger mentions the variety of units (including 'half *clepsydrae*') asked for and allotted to litigants. It is Pliny, too, who gives our best evidence for the relationship of the legal *clepsydra* unit to the hour, in a rare instance of a text which mentions both kinds of measurement in tandem. He says that in a particular legal context he spoke for nearly five hours, and relates this to the number of *clepsydrae* he was given, namely sixteen. The *clepsydra* length thus seems to be roughly fifteen minutes.[19]

Accuracy

We thus have two main mechanisms of time measurement. But what guarantees the accuracy, in either case? And how important an issue was this felt to be? Certainly, the problem of accuracy of sundials is one which is raised occasionally in our extant texts, as for example in Seneca's famous remark that it is easier to find agreement between philosophers than between sundials, or in the Elder Pliny's observation that the first sundial erected at the Rostra was inaccurate (but nevertheless obeyed).[20] But we find almost no discussion, either of the principles

---

18 Conflicts would arise, also, in this Roman judicial context, between the competing authorities of judge and clock: see Ker (2009); Riggsby (2009).
19 Cicero's remark is at *On the Orator* 3.138 ('hunc non clamator aliqui ad clepsydram latrare docuerat ... sed Anaxagoras, vir summus in maximarum rerum scientia', 'it was not some bawler who had taught him [Pericles] to bark against the clock, but ... Anaxagoras, a man outstanding for his knowledge of the highest matters'); cf. *Tusculan Disputations* 2.67. At *Letters* 6.2.5 Pliny mentions the current custom of allotting units as short as half a *clepsydra*. His account of the length of a speech of his own, and its relationship to actual hours, is at *Letters* 2.11.14–16: 'dixi horis paene quinque, nam duodecim clepsydris, quas spatiosissimas accepi, sunt additae quattuor ...' I give the length in minutes as calculated by Wolkenhauer (2020: 228), who takes into account the time of year of the speech (implying that a 50-minute hour was in question) and the fact that Pliny characterizes the first 12 *clepsydrae* he was given as particularly full.
20 Seneca, *Apocolyntosis* 2.2 ('facilius inter philosophos quam inter horologia conveniet'); Pliny, *Natural History* 7.60.214. (Pliny here mentions the gratitude with which the erection of the improved sundial was received, 99 years later, and also the value of a water-based mechanism, dedicated indoors in 159 BCE, in improving the accuracy of time measurement visible to the public.) There is scholarly discussion as to whether the inaccuracy of this early sundial in the forum was due to its original construction for the different latitude of Catania, or its poor design; for an analysis of the effects of such displacement on the instrument's accuracy, see the detailed

and methods of construction of sundials, or of the question of the agreement or non-agreement *between* these two technologies of time measurement.

In fact, a text by the philosophical and medical author Galen, in the late second century CE, seems to provide us with a unique case where both these problems are directly addressed. As is so often the case with this author's insights, the remarks in question are quite tangential to the main purpose and argumentative context of the text in which they appear, which is the treatise entitled *Affections and Errors of the Soul*. In the second part of this work, aimed at eradicating errors (*hamartēmata*) of human reasoning, Galen inveighs against professional or self-styled philosophers who engage in debates on unanswerable metaphysical questions, and also against those who engage in debates on important matters without an elementary logical training or an understanding of what constitutes a demonstrative or scientific argument. He points to mathematics and geometry as paradigmatic disciplines for the kind of argument, and the kind of logical training, he has in mind. The crucial feature of these disciplines is that their results 'provide their own confirmation to those who find them out'. They are, that is to say, self-confirming: one who arrives at the correct answer in these areas cannot doubt that it has been arrived at. Earlier in the treatise, before the passage that we shall now look at in detail, he has given as examples of such 'self-confirming' procedures the division of a line into equal sections, the drawing of a circle around a given square (or vice versa), or the same operation with a circle and a number of other equiangular polygons.[21]

But the example of mathematical and geometrical procedure that he elaborates on at length is that of the design and construction of a sundial. The passage is of interest to us from a number of points of view, and I therefore quote it *in extenso*.

> Imagine that a city is being founded, and that the prospective inhabitants want to know, not roughly but with precision, on each and every day, how much of the time has passed, and how much is left, before sunset. According to the method of *analysis*, this problem must be referred to the first *kritērion*, if one wishes to find it out in the manner we learned in the study [or treatise] of gnomons; one must then go down the same path in the opposite direction to put the solution together [*suntithenai*, cognate with *synthesis*], again as we learned in that same study. When we have in this way found the path that is to be followed in all cases, and once we have realized that this kind of measurement of periods of time

---

discussion of Jones (2020: 137–43). It seems also from archaeological evidence that many sundials, e. g. the large number found at Pompeii and Herculaneum, were quite inaccurate; see Wolkenhauer (2020: 234, n. 53), with further literature there cited; but this is of course a different matter from there being a contemporary *awareness* of this inaccuracy.

21 Galen, *Affections and Errors* 2.3, 46–7 De Boer (V.66–8 K.).

within the day must be carried out by means of geometric lines, we must then proceed to the materials which will receive the imprint [*or* drawing] of the lines, and the gnomon. And first we must enquire which shapes of bodies will be suitable for the design which we have found out; then we must find out in each case, by *analysis* and *synthesis*, how the design should be done; then, whenever the method of logic indicates to us that there are manifest grounds for trust in the discovery of the matters before us, we must then turn to the practical realization of the things discovered by it, and, again, examine how we are to produce a flat surface for the body to be drawn. And once we have found this out by *analysis* and *synthesis*, and have constructed some such body, we must find out which instruments should be used to draw it; and when, once again, this has been discovered by *analysis* and *synthesis*, we must attempt to construct them in the form taught to us by the method. Then, we must make a series of drawings in many forms and give them to people to test in practice whether the task set has been accomplished. For when the first line is hit by the first ray of the sun, and in the same manner the last by the last, and when this is apparent in the case of all the drawn [lines of the] sundials, we will then in a way have one manifest indicator that the problem set has been found out. Another consists in the fact that the lines drawn are all in agreement with each other ...[22]

A couple of things here require comment before we go any further. One is that the text of the passage is uncertain in some details: both this and the one which we shall look at next are particularly beset with textual difficulties, even within a text which in general has a problematic manuscript tradition.[23] A second is the conceptual background implied by the repeated terminology of *analysis* and *synthesis*. These are terms ultimately from the Platonist philosophical tradition, though also used in reference to the solution of geometrical problems. The fundamental notion is that of an interlocking operation of two procedures, which as it were go in opposite directions. *Analysis* is literally a 'solving upwards', a procedure of making reference to the fundamental principles or axioms which apply to the problem (principles or axioms referred to here by the term *kritērion*). *Synthesis* is a procedure literally of 'putting together', by which is understood the application of the principles just mentioned to the particular case or instantiation of the problem, or to its different parts.

All that said, there is tantalizingly little information, in concrete detail, as to precisely what Galen has in mind in his description of each stage of the process; one is, indeed, tempted to say that he is engaging in a good deal of 'hand-wav-

---

22 Galen, *Affections and Errors* 2.5, 54–5 De Boer (V.80–2 K.), trans. Singer (2013): 299–300.
23 It is a curiosity of the history of scholarship on ancient medical texts that these passages were the first in the treatise to receive modern scholarly attention; this was from Joachim Marquardt in 1865, who evidently thought their understanding to be the most urgent issue, and devoted a publication to this part of the text before a critical edition of the whole treatise had been attempted. A first such edition was then produced by his own son, Johannes, in 1884.

ing'. Particularly tantalizing is the reference to a *pragmateia* ('study' or 'treatise') on gnomons, with which he suggests that he (and possibly his imagined addressee, depending on whether we take the 'we' here as literal or 'royal') are familiar. It is almost certainly relevant here that Galen's father is known to have been an architect or civil engineer – *architektōn*, a practitioner of *architektonia* – and that it is to the discipline of *architektonia* that, as Galen points out, this procedure belongs. While it is frustrating that the reference to a detailed treatise on the subject seems to take the place of any clear account of the actual mathematics, it is nevertheless of interest that Galen claims to have consulted such a work, and seems to think it not an unreasonable expectation that his reader could get hold of one. Our reflections above regarding the status of sundials as related to the high-status notion of Greek *paideia* may be pertinent here too: the *aspiration* to participate in the knowledge or wisdom related to the sun, the heavenly bodies and time may be a significant social or cultural factor. This consideration does not, of course, enable us to answer the question, how widespread was a genuine technical knowledge or detailed understanding of the relevant scientific or mathematical principles.[24]

Moreover, however skimpy on technical detail, the passage is of considerable value in relation to our previous discussion, both in confirming and in filling out the picture that has emerged so far. First, the suggestion at the very beginning of the passage that the people of a city would want to be able to monitor the passing of the hours 'not roughly but with precision' is relevant to our understanding of ancient attitudes to time measurement; we shall return to this question of precision a little later. Secondly, and consistently with what we know from the archaeological evidence mentioned above, Galen mentions a variety of possible shapes as suitable for the instantiation of the design – even though he does seem to end up with a flat surface as the core example upon which he focuses.[25]

Then, he mentions the obvious requirement of the sun's shadow hitting the different lines at the right moments as one criterion of success, and the slightly less obvious one of the lines being 'in agreement with each other' – presumably a criterion of symmetry, although again there is a lack of detail, and one would

---

24 On Galen's father, cf. n. 10 above. As pointed out to me by Kassandra Miller, what Galen has in mind with his mention of a *pragmateia* concerning gnomons may possibly be the same thing referred to by both Vitruvius (9.1.1) and Ptolemy as an *analēmma*, that is a diagram enabling the maker of a clock to proceed on the basis of the right grid. Those texts, too, however, fail to give further detail of the *analēmmata* themselves, nor, of course, do they help us know how widespread would have been their circulation.

25 For the full range of possible designs see Jones (2020).

need to add mathematical precision to make such a symmetry criterion a valid one.

In fact, though, his mention of that first requirement – obvious though indeed it is – raises more questions than it answers. Apart from the moments of sunrise and sunset, and perhaps that of midday, *how* will the observer know that the hour lines have been drawn in the right places?

But it is precisely here that Galen introduces his clearest and most interesting insight into the question of time measurement – one indeed that is unique in ancient literature. The text continues.

> ... and a third [manifest indicator that the problem set has been solved consists] in the confirmation by an even flow of water, for the argument discovers that this, too, will be a *kritērion* of the correctness of the sundials drawn. Let me explain what I mean. Make a hole in a vessel, which may be of any material you wish, and place it in clear water at the moment when you see the first ray of the sun. Then, when the sundial that has been drawn indicates the completion of the first hour, make a mark in the vessel at the point to which it has been filled by the water; then empty it immediately and replace it in the same water. When the sundial reports the second hour, examine the vessel; then, once you find that the water in it has reached the same point that you marked at the first hour, again quickly empty it and replace in in the same place in the water. Examine it again, and see if the sundial indicates that the water has reached the same point in the third hour that it did in the first and the second ... Once you find that the water has reached the same place in this hour too, and then also in the sixth, and also in each of the subsequent hours up to the twelfth, you will be convinced – unless you are entirely lacking in understanding – that the sundial was properly designed, since, indeed, it has displayed the matter before us. And the matter before us was the division of the day into twelve equal parts.[26]

The notion of the interacting observations of water-flow and progress of the sun to arrive at, or correct, the drawing of sundial lines on the ground provides a fascinating, and unique, example of the use of such a confirmatory procedure in this context. Other texts, such as those cited above which complain of the inaccuracy of sundials, give no indication of the criteria by which such a conclusion has been reached. And the only other text which makes a direct equivalence between 'hour' time and *clepsydra* time, that of Pliny, is not talking about confirmation, nor, indeed, referring to any particular way of measuring the hours in question.

It is important to note here, however, that Galen is not talking about a water-clock or *clepsydra* in the usual sense. The particular procedure he mentions combines an essential feature of the forensic-context *clepsydra* (restriction to measurement of a single block of time) with an essential feature of the sophisticated

---

[26] Galen, *Affections and Errors* 2.5, 55–6 De Boer (V.82–3 K.), trans. Singer (2013): 300–1.

subdivided-vessel *clepsydrae* (that it involves a constant inflow of water); however, it is neither of these things, but rather an ad hoc testing mechanism designed for a particular purpose. Again with Galen's personal connection to the profession of *architektōn* in mind, it is tempting to think that such a procedure may indeed have been used to adjust or correct sundials during construction.[27]

But Galen is not finished yet. For he does indeed proceed to describe the design of a water-clock – which again he claims to be an example of 'the method of *analysis*'. Here, too, we experience the same frustration as in the first passage, both as regards what precisely is meant by *analysis* and as regards the actual procedure. Even more so, indeed: Galen makes no attempt at all to describe the mathematical *procedure* by which the clock is constructed or the lines on it drawn, but only the final layout and function of those lines once successfully completed.[28] The passage is nevertheless of interest as a thorough account of such a *clepsydra*, designed to record the passing of the hours accurately on each day of the year. (See figure 6.)

> Thus, too, reason, conducting its enquiry by the method of *analysis*, has found out the design of the water-clock – where, again, the test of its correctness is something manifest even to the layman. Here, the uppermost line, that which indicates the twelfth hour of the day, is at its highest in that part of the water-clock which measures the longest day, and at its lowest in that part which measures the shortest; midway between these two is the marker corresponding to the equinoxes. The area between these divisions, on the lip of the water-clock, indicates to you the days after these four. Starting from these divisions, you will find, next after the marker which represents the longest day, that which indicates the point on the top line which the water will reach on completion of the twelfth hour on the following day. And again, the third along from the solstice will indicate to you the third day, and the next the fourth day. And, carrying on in the same way, you will find that every day of the year is marked by this one line in the water-clock which I have said is the uppermost. The other lines, meanwhile, which are lower than this highest one, you will find measure out the other hours: the first one down from the 'twelfth' represents the eleventh hour – at a different point on it for each day of the year (in exactly the same way as we just explained in the case of the uppermost line); the next after that indicates the tenth hour, similarly, at different points along it; the one after that, again,

---

[27] It should be noted, however, alongside what was said above about the simple outflow device standardly used in the Athenian law court, that we also have evidence for a simple, non-subdivided, *inflow* device. The *clepsydra* described by Simplicius, *On Aristotle's On the Heavens* 2.13, 524,19–25 Heiberg, as discussed by Hannah (2009: 100), is a perforated vessel which is submerged in water, and then takes a fixed time to fill up. This is somewhat similar to what is here described by Galen.

[28] Such descriptions are extremely rare; an attempt (vitiated by errors) to give the relevant measurements appears on a papyrus, *P. Oxy.* 470.31–85, translated and discussed by Sherwood et al. (2020): 627–8.

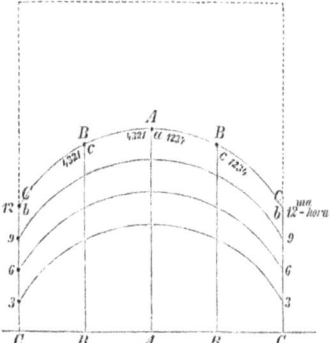

Figure 6: Diagram of Galen's account of the design of a water-clock. The diagram, showing the varying length of the vertical lines corresponding to hours at different seasons, is based on the description at *Affections and Errors* 2.5, and is taken from Marquardt et al. (1884), p. XX.

the ninth; then the eighth, and so on, down to the lowest line, which finds out the first hours, just as it appears on the sundials; and as the level of the water in the water-clock rises, the first and indeed all following hours appear equal, right up to the twelfth; but not equal to those on the preceding and following days.[29]

The fact that Galen describes this object in detail suggests that it was one which his reader might encounter, either in a public space or at least in a private dwelling. It is worth noting, too, that in spite of the theoretical capacity, mentioned above, of water-clocks to measure much shorter timespans than that of an hour, Galen has no such expectation for the water-clock which he describes in detail here; rather, it seems to function simply as an alternative to the sundial. Another feature of the use of the object is of interest, too: unlike the case with a sundial, the reader of this device must know in advance what day of the year it is in order to follow the upward vertical path of the water at the right horizontal position on the vessel. Finally, the passage is of interest also for the question of the nature of confirmation, although it again does not answer it. Indeed, the nature of the confirmation in this case – the process by which the 'correctness' is 'manifest even to the layman' – is not made explicit. Presumably, though

---

29 Galen, *Affections and Errors* 2.5, 57–8 De Boer (V.84–6 K.), trans. Singer (2013): 302–3; and for discussion of the design Galen is describing, see the note by Singer (2013) ad loc.: 302–3, n. 107. It is essential – since what is at issue is still the accurate measurement of *seasonal* hours – that while the inflow to the device is constant, there must be a system of calibration that marks the hours differentially on different days. Further on seasonal hours, see below, pp. 31–3.

(and as perhaps suggested by the phrase 'just as it appears on the sundials'), the confirmation Galen has in mind is indeed that through a sundial – one which has been correctly constructed as confirmed by the previous procedure. We thus have an intriguing – and, in the literature, unique – account of ancient perceptions of accuracy in the measurement of time, and, even more specifically, of the mutually interactive way in which the accuracy of the available time devices was assessed.[30]

Time perception, time management and the use of time-telling devices

Some of the questions considered above are largely technical in nature. But they lead us on to the consideration of other questions, of a social-historical or even psychological nature. How aware were people of the passing of the hours, or of 'what time' it was at any given moment? How important a part of everyday life was the precise measurement of time? In what contexts – by whom, and for what specific purposes – were the sophisticated instruments of time measurement available to the Romans actually used? How important was accuracy of time measurement, and relatedly promptness, in Roman society?

Our first passage from Galen above already gave one perspective on the first question – the perceived civic need for accurate measurement of the hours. And archaeological evidence suggests an increasingly prominent role for time-telling devices in public spaces – including in some cases water-clocks – in the Roman imperial period; locations where some kind of public clock was on display included fora, gymnasia, theatres and sanctuaries.[31] Still, the picture is a mixed one, and one might doubt, on the basis of other texts, how deeply such a need was felt, or how precise such measurement needed to be.

---

30 But there is *some* other literary evidence of the use of the one kind of technology as a check on the other: Cicero tell of bored participants at the lawcourts sending a slave out to check the hour, presumably on a sundial (*Brutus* 200). Julius Caesar's report of his expedition's discovery in Britain, 'by precise water measurements, that the nights are shorter than on the continent' ('certis ex aqua mensuris breviores esse quam in continenti', *Gallic War* 5.13.4), i.e. by some form of water-clock, is also in some sense an attempt to improve on the accuracy of what was known on the basis of the observation of the sun.

31 For comprehensive lists of such locations see Winter (2013), vol. 2: 195–215. Some form of water-clock is attested, in Galen's own time, for a theatre at Priene and both a *gumnasion* and an *agora* at Pergamum. But in all contexts, public and private, remains of sundials greatly outnumber those of water-clocks.

Several Roman literary authors mention the division of the day into hours in the context of their own individual accounts of the way in which their day is spent, or their organization of time within the day.³² In such accounts, periods smaller than that of an hour are never mentioned. But even the division of the day into hours is often approximate; many activities go over more than one hour, or are allotted vaguely to one hour or another; and it is also a feature of such accounts that only a few specific hours are mentioned. As a generalization, explicit references to hours of the morning are much more frequent than references to those of the latter half of the day.³³

So, for example, Pliny the Younger's account of his scheme of organization of leisured days at his Tuscan villa makes explicit mention only of the first and the fourth or fifth hours, and adds that even here the measures are not exact in relation to his actual activities.

> I wake up ... about the first hour, often earlier ... When I am working on something, I think about it word by word ... I call for the notary and dictate what I have produced, after the light of the day has been allowed to enter ... When the fourth or fifth hour comes (there is no set or fixed time), I move to the terrace or portico ... I think over and dictate the rest. I get into a carriage. There I keep doing the same thing that I have been doing while walking and lying down; my attention is maintained and animated by the change. I sleep a little, then go for a walk, then read a Greek or Latin speech aloud, with concentration, more for the sake of my stomach than for that of my voice ... I then walk again; have myself oiled; exercise; bathe. During dinner ... I have a book read to me; after dinner there is a comedy or a lyre-player; then I walk with my associates, who include educated people. Thus the evening continues in varied conversation, and even the longest day is well concluded.³⁴

He adds, finally, that the above scheme admits of a degree of variation in detail.

Cicero's somewhat similar, but more melancholic, account of his life of retreat after the end of the Civil War is vague, especially in relation to the later parts of the day. After a certain point in the day – but he does not specify which point – all his time is given over to the body ('inde corpori omne tempus

---

32 For such discussions and for more detail of such texts see Ker (2020); Wolkenhauer (2020). Both Martial, *Epigrams* 8.67.1 and Juvenal, *Satires* 10.216, make reference to the practice of slave boy announcing the time of day to his master; the passages are discussed by Hannah (2009): 105.
33 This bias is arguably, however, a function of the particular context, namely that of texts that focus on literary or intellectual activity; in the different context of the gymnasium, of course, precise times might be allotted to a variety of activities and procedures. There is, moreover, some inscriptional evidence of precise times being allotted, differentially to men and women, for their activities within the gymnasium. I am grateful to Kassandra Miller for both these observations.
34 Pliny, *Letters* 9.36.1–5

datur'). He is, however, clearer about the order and timing of activities in the morning, which begins with the *salutatio*, continues with time spent on his *litterae* (that is, on writing or reading).[35]

It should be observed that the above two examples, in their different ways, both reflect a life of rural retreat, which is in some respects to be contrasted with – and in Roman literature often is explicitly contrasted with – the life of the city. Some basic structural similarities, however, seem to apply to both, in particular the expectation that some form of business and literary activities will occupy the morning hours, and some combination of physical exercise and cultural or leisure activities the afternoon and evening ones.

Even Martial's well-known 'hour epigram', which is deliberately, and doubtless artificially, precise about hours, as a function of the literary conceit it is attempting, has considerable fuzziness: the first and second hours are again occupied in the *salutatio*, the third in lawsuits; but from then until the fifth there can be a variety of tasks or duties, and the rest that comes around the sixth hour is somewhat vague as to its precise extent. Exercise will occupy the eighth and ninth hours, after which dinner fades into the *hora libellorum meorum*, which is presumably an extension of it, and no hour is mentioned after the tenth.[36]

Certainly, a pattern of elite time organization emerges from all this. To simplify, this tends to involve meeting and greeting associates, patrons or clients, as the first activity in the morning, followed by attention to business, legal, or literary activity; and there is usually some form of exercise or other relaxation after midday, whether this is simply passive exercise in a carriage, alongside some vocalization, or actual *palaestra* exercise. This relaxation or exercise regime is sometimes described as 'time devoted to the body', a phrase which we shall find echoed and reinforced in Galen's medical discourse. And indeed, such a pattern is related to the more detailed patterns of exercise regime mentioned by Galen in the medical context, as we shall see shortly.

How important actual time measurement, that is, consultation of a time-telling device of some sort, whether sun- or water-based, was to the conduct or organization of such daily activities – even in cases where the activities *are* delimited in terms of hours, as they are, albeit partially, in the examples given above – is difficult to determine on the basis of our literary evidence. The practice of Spurinna, who had an attendant inform him, presumably on the basis of observation of some time-telling device, of the correct time to bathe each day, is men-

---

35 Cicero, *Letters to Friends* 9.20.3.
36 Martial, *Epigrams* 4.8.

tioned with approval by Pliny the Younger;[37] and Galen's evidence certainly seems to imply that elite Romans did pay attention to the precise hour in the organization of their exercise activity. There is also some evidence of resistance to the regulation of the day by the division into hours by the sundial, for example in a fragment of Plautus relayed by Aulus Gellius. The context is a comic one, where the speaker complains of a town full of people shrivelled up by hunger because they are not allowed to eat until the sun allows it; but it suggests that the domination of the 'new' technology was felt as an unwelcome intrusion, or even tyranny, by some.[38]

The related question arises of promptness, which is discussed in an illuminating way by Wolkenhauer (2020). As she points out, while there is certainly a strong notion developed in Roman society of lateness, or coming too late for an appointment, this is understood in terms of missing an opportunity for action, and the lateness never defined in terms of an actual time on the clock.

Medical texts and practices concerning time management

Whether the insistence on precise hours implies a close reliance on time-telling devices, specifically on the part of *medical* practitioners, is again a difficult question to answer. Clearly, texts which insist either on activities being performed, or on diagnostic indicators being observed, at a particular hour, imply that the doctor believes himself to have some accurate, and readily available, way of determining those hours. The actual technology used is, however, not explicitly mentioned. Here reference should however be made to two pieces of evidence which may suggest the use, by a doctor, of portable time-telling devices.

One is the archaeological find, amongst a set of medical instruments, of an artefact which has been interpreted by some scholars as a portable sundial. The other, which we will consider in more detail in the last chapter, is the use, attributed to Herophilus, of a portable water-clock to determine the frequency of the pulse. It should, however, be emphasized that both these pieces of evidence are, to say the least, inconclusive. In the former case, the function of the object can-

---

37 *Letters* 3.1. The disparaging remark of Seneca, meanwhile, about those who have to be reminded when to wash, swim or dine (*The Shortness of Life* 12.6), seems directed rather at a certain kind of pampered idleness than at the practice of paying attention to the clock. Both passages are discussed by Hannah (2009): 105. For further discussion of the question of the requirement of accurate time measurement in Roman life see Talbert (2020).
38 Aulus Gellius, *Attic Nights* 3.3.5.

not be determined with certainty; in the latter, the report is from a single source, writing probably several centuries after Herophilus, and presenting the account as an anecdote. And even if we take both as completely reliable pieces of evidence, they are wholly isolated ones, which can hardly be used to extrapolate a general picture of ancient medical practice.[39]

It is, however, in medical texts that we find the most detailed concern with regulation according to hours.

Medical prescriptions, both those for normal daily regime in cases of health and those involving one-off interventions in the case of sickness, frequently specify precise times of day. Many examples could be given, especially of the latter, pathological, context. Here we move into the complex area of periodic illnesses, and the intricacies surrounding the calculation of their precise hour of recurrence, and the appropriate interventions to be given – or avoided – at those times. This topic which will be considered in more detail in chapter 4. Let a couple of examples suffice, from Galen's vivid autobiographical account of his clinical interactions with the imperial family, *Prognosis*.

> What was genuinely remarkable was what happened in the case of the emperor himself at this time. Both he and those doctors in his entourage who had travelled with him on campaign believed that he was experiencing the onset of the episode of a fever, but all were misled, as shown on the second and third days, both in the morning and at the eighth hour. On the previous day he had taken the aloe-based bitter medicine at the first hour, followed by theriac – which he took as part of his daily routine – around the sixth hour. He had then bathed around sunset, and taken a little nourishment. Throughout the night he experienced stomach cramps, as well as the voiding of his bowel, as a result of which he began to run a fever. The doctors in his entourage, on examining him first thing in the morning, ordered him to rest, then gave him some gruel to eat at the ninth hour. After this I was myself summoned to sleep in the Palace; and it was shortly after the lighting of the lamps that someone was sent to me from the emperor. Now, since there were three doctors who had already seen him, both in the morning and around the eighth hour, and all had taken his pulse and discerned the onset of an episode, I stood still and said nothing; so that it was the emperor who looked at me and initiated the interrogation. Why, he asked, had I, alone of the doctors, not made an investigation by touch?[40]

Galen feigns reluctance to intervene, on the grounds that the other doctors who have attended the emperor know his constitution better and should be better placed to advise and predict. When finally pressed to take the emperor's

---

39 On the 'Este Dial' (a cylindrical tube found at the 'tomb of the physician' at Palazzina Capodaglio, near Este, in 1901) and its interpretation see Bonomi (1984); Arnaldi and Schaldach (1997). For Marcellinus on Herophilus see below, p. 160.
40 Galen, *Prognosis* 11, 126–8 Nutton (XIV.657–9 K.). The episode is depicted in figure 12 below.

pulse, he ventures the view that there is no onset of fever, but merely a problem of digestion.

A little later in the work, he recounts the complimentary remarks made to him – or rather, made about him to his rival Methodists doctors – by the lady Annia Faustina, after his successful treatment of the boy Commodus, who had become feverish after a session in the gymnasium:

> 'You should know that Galen, here, combats you Methodists not with words but with deeds. He has frequently before now prescribed bathing for people beginning a fever, and given them wine to drink; and he has allowed some to return to their usual activities on the first day, others on the third. You, meanwhile, all instruct them in all cases to fast for the first two days, and to remain lying down until the suspected hours have passed. So now he has shown the reliability of his knowledge, when the son of the emperor, in his father's absence, had a violent fever on the first two days – as you yourselves heard yesterday – yet on the third day he did not wait for the eighth hour to pass, as you think right, but prescribed bathing and nourishment. And even his tutor, Peitholaus, who is such a careful man in such matters that his care may seem to be timidity, was persuaded, by his previous experience of the man's skill, to allow washing and feeding before the suspected hour.'[41]

Both passages thoroughly exemplify the centrality of precise hours of the day to the Roman medical discourse, diagnostically and therapeutically. Food, rest and medicine are prescribed for particular hours; the 'suspected' hour of onset of an episodic fever is awaited, and certain interventions avoided just before it. And we note that such time measurement is equally important both to Galen – the precise details of whose analysis of periodicity we shall explore further in chapter 4 – and to his arch-rivals, the Methodists, who insist on a three-day period of fasting in response to almost all disease conditions.

The use of specific times of day is a prominent feature of the prescription or description of daily regimes for states of health, too. Parallels could also be given for the classical Greek period – with the proviso stated above, that in the former case the times of day in question are not analysed in terms of numerical hours.[42] Let us consider two examples from the Roman imperial period, given by Galen in his major work on health.

> The safest procedure, in the case of weak old men, is to give little food, three times a day. This is the daily regime that the doctor Antiochus imposed upon himself; and he reached an age of more than eighty years, going every day to the public forum, to the place where the citizens' council chamber itself was, and sometimes also making a long journey out of

---

41 Galen, *Prognosis* 12, 132 Nutton (XIV.663–4 K.)
42 See e.g. the detailed discussion of exercise regimes in relation to times of day and meal times at 'Hippocrates', *Regimen* 3.68.

town to examine a patient. He used to make the journey from his house to the public forum – a distance of roughly three *stadia* – on foot, and in this way too he would visit those patients who lived nearby. If he was ever compelled to make a longer journey, he would do so either in a litter or in a carriage. There was a room in his house which was heated by a furnace in winter, but had well-mixed air, even without a fire, in summer. It was here that he would always undergo massage, both in winter and in summer – after first defaecating, of course. At the place to which he went in the forum, he would eat bread with Attic honey, around the third, or at the latest the fourth, hour; the honey would usually be cooked, but occasionally raw. He would then continue up to the seventh hour either engaging others in discussion, or reading alone, after which he would spend time in the public bath house, and perform the exercises appropriate for an old man, the nature of which will be stated a little later. Then, after bathing, he would have his lunch, which would be a well-balanced one: first, he would take those things that empty the stomach, and after that mainly fish – both those of rocky water and those of deep water. Then, at dinner, he would refrain from the consumption of fish, but would take those foods which have the best fluid and which are not prone to decay: groats with wine-honey, or a bird cooked in a simple sauce.

By applying this old-age care to himself, Antiochus continued right to the end with his senses unimpaired and his limbs supple. Telephus the scholar reached an even greater age than Antiochus, living nearly 100 years. He would bathe twice a month in the winter, four times in the summer and three times in the intervening seasons. On days when he did not bathe, he would have oil applied around the third hour, with a short massage. He would then eat groats boiled in water, with the addition of the finest raw honey: this would be sufficient for him for his first meal. He, too, would have his lunch at the seventh hour, or a little earlier, taking vegetables first and then enjoying birds or fish. In the evening he would eat bread alone, soaking it in diluted wine.[43]

Again, the text is remarkable for the detail given of both diet and other daily activities, all tied to precise times of the day. And we find some evidence that such daily regimes were taken seriously in non-medical literature too: Pliny the Younger's account of the regime of baths, exercise and other daily activity undergone by the 77-year-old Spurinna provides a quite close parallel to the above – not, to be sure, in the details of the prescriptions (Spurinna bathes daily, though at different times in summer and winter, and undertakes a seven-mile carriage ride as well as exercise with a ball), but in the attention to the correct time, nature and quantity of the relevant elements: baths, exercise, rest.[44]

Let us turn, finally, to an example which casts light both on the organization of time as related to the maintenance of a healthy lifestyle and on anxieties that might arise in this context. The passage also returns us to the issues we considered earlier, of the variable hours in use in Roman time-keeping, and of the awareness of the passing of time in relation to these.

---

43 Galen, *Health* 5.4, 143–4 Koch (VI.332–4 K.)
44 Pliny, *Letters* 3.1.

The first focus of this discussion will be the person with a bodily constitution which is faultless ... but with a life of servitude, involving service to a monarch or person of great power throughout the whole day, but some freedom from this service at either end of it. But here too we must clarify what is meant by 'end': without some appropriate specification the term may lead to misunderstanding on the part of the reader. If I state that someone has the freedom to attend to the care of his body once the sun sets, without adding which day is in question – whether it is near to the summer or winter solstice, or to one of the equinoxes, or at one of the midpoints between these – then it will be impossible to offer the appropriate precepts. In Rome, for example, the longest days and nights are slightly more than fifteen equinoctial hours in length, while the shortest ones are slightly less than nine. In Alexandria, on the other hand, the longest are fourteen and the shortest ten. Now, when the days are shortest, and the nights longest, someone whose duties end at sunset will easily be able to undergo massage and bathing, and to take a balanced amount of sleep; but one who is in the same situation when the [days] are longest will not be able to carry out even one of these activities to the right degree. But I have not yet known one whose personal circumstances were as unfortunate as that.

Indeed, the emperor who was keenest to attend to the care of his body (amongst those I have known) was Marcus Aurelius. He would go to the wrestling school at sunset on short days, but at the ninth or at the latest the tenth hour on the longest days, so that it was possible those who accompanied him throughout his daily activities to retire and take care of their bodies during the remaining part of the day, and then to go to bed at sunset.[45] (The shortest night, being equal in length to nine equinoctial hours, would provide them with sufficient sleep.)[46]

Galen refers to an ideal here, that of having 'leisure for the body alone'. The life of leisure, or more precisely the life free of public obligations or work constraints, is frequently mentioned throughout this text as representing the optimal circumstance, from which other forms of life are departures. Temporal freedom – the power to dispose of one's own time as one wishes – is both a crucial demarcator of an elite lifestyle, and potentially of crucial importance to health. Galen wants to insist, however, that a healthy regime may be pursued, in spite of limitations on this freedom, precisely by dint of good time management. In that sense, Galen's model seems largely compatible with those implied by the Latin literary texts considered above. Even if one only finds a certain part of the day, after the end of one's other duties, to devote 'to the body alone', this may be sufficient. As we saw above, such a model of relaxation in the afternoon, of a distinct – or rather, a flexible – time available for one's exercise, after the

---

45 Sunset on the shortest day of all in Rome would fall at about 16.40; the ninth hour at the summer solstice would fall at roughly 16.55, and the tenth at 18.10. For another ancient discussion of the differences of daylight hours at different latitudes, calculated in equinoctial hours, see Pliny, *Natural History* 2.77.186–7.
46 Galen, *Health* 6.5, 178–9 Koch (VI.404–6 K.).

termination of one's more pressing duties, is evidenced in other authors too; and indeed we observed a closely similar notion, 'from this point all the time is given to my body', in Cicero. It is interesting also to note the specific reference to the *tenth* hour as the latest moment that members of the emperor's entourage would be released. This seems to echo Seneca's observation about the orator Asinius Pollio, 'the great orator who was never detained by any matter beyond the tenth hour'.[47] Marcus Aurelius on Galen's account is complying with a broadly traditional, or perhaps better a civilized Roman, understanding of the 'work–life balance'.

Perhaps ironically, one of the few texts which we have which complains of the problems of maintaining such a 'work–life balance', or of keeping to an exercise regime in spite of one's duties, does not come from an emperor's servant but from an emperor himself. According to Suetonius, the emperor Augustus wrote to Tiberius as follows:

> Not even a Jew on the Sabbath fasts so rigorously as I did today: I managed to grab a couple of mouthfuls in the bathing house, after the first hour of the night, just before I began my massage.[48]

A further point of interest arising from the Galenic text just considered is that of the relationship between seasonal and equinoctial hours. We have observed the prevalent role of the seasonal hours in this culture, as a function of ancient methods of time measurement. Yet the above text shows Galen fully aware of the number of *equinoctial* hours to which longer or shorter days correspond, in each case; and indeed he suggests that the emperor's own daily schedule actually followed a timetable which could be better analysed in terms of the latter than of the former. That is, he goes to the gymnasium at roughly the same time, *in modern terms*, all the year round: 16.40 (sunset on the shortest day) or 16.55 (ninth hour on the longest) – although admittedly the possibility of the tenth hour in the latter case takes us as late as 18.10. The text thus raises some interesting – though perhaps unanswerable – questions, in terms of the relationship between the two in most people's minds. To what extent were people in general

---

[47] Seneca, *Tranquility of Mind* 17.7 ('oratorem magnum ... quem nulla res ultra decumam detinuit'). The broader context is, again, the ethical importance of the division, traditionally instituted, between periods of work and periods of leisure. In the same passage Seneca also remarks that no motion is allowed in the senate after the tenth hour.

[48] Suetonius, *Augustus* 76.2 ('ne Iudaeus quidem ... tam diligenter sabbatis ieiunium servat quam ego hodie servavi, qui in balineo demum post horam primam noctis duas buccas manducavi priusquam ungui inciperem').

aware of the fixed hours lying behind the seasonal ones that they had, for official and practical purposes, to deal with? Were others – as Galen is here – inclined to make the mental conversion between the two? And if so, how easy or accessible was such a conversion for most people?

Galen against 'festive time'

Finally, in relation to Galen's medical or healthful regulation of the day, it is interesting to note the negative remarks he makes in this connection regarding people's behaviour on public holidays. I do not enter here into the larger question of the differential perception of 'festive time' in premodern societies, which has been discussed by a number of scholars.[49] It seems, however, that the Galenic medical model in a strong sense explicitly *excludes* such differential experience of festive time – that it constitutes, indeed, an alternative model, according to which divisions of the year or month due to human convention or religious observation are actively to be rejected, insofar as they might have a significant effect on human behaviour. Rather, Galen aims to subsume 'festive' time within the domain of 'normal' time: specifically, he regards the former as an opportunity to continue and indeed extend the healthy *diaita* that one has been practising within the latter. As he comments:

> People could, in fact, make such provision for themselves, on days when there is some public festival, which frees them from their servitude; but because of their lack of restraint they not only do nothing to correct such accumulation in the body, but actually exacerbate the situation by their bad regime on those occasions.[50]

For Galen and the medical discourse that he champions there are, to be sure, special days and hours – moments to which one should attribute a particular significance, or treat in a special way. But – as we have seen above in the context of hours, and will see further in chapter 4 in the context of both hours and days within the month – this 'special' status is given by natural cycles, cycles which are a function of human nature, the nature of one's environment, or of the cosmos, not by arbitrary or god-given calendrical observations.

This is a medical and ethical discourse which aims to exert its control, not just over the whole lived day, but also over the whole lived year, abolishing any

---

49 On the Roman calendar in its social dimension see Rüpke (1995), (2011); Hannah (2005), ch. 5; and for one specific analysis Beard (1987).
50 Galen, *Health* 6.7, 182 Koch (VI.415 K.).

conceptual difference between normal (official, business or commercial) and festive time. As we shall see in the next chapter, it also exerts its control over every successive season, and every time of life.

Chapter Two:
Times of life and times of year: the ever-shifting cycles

Introductory

In this chapter I explore two kinds of cycle, both of fundamental importance for people's perception and understanding of time in relation to their everyday existence: life cycles and the yearly cycle of the seasons. As in the previous chapter, we shall begin with a consideration of the broader Graeco-Roman background, before homing in on the theories, perceptions of life experience, and practical interventions found in specifically medical texts. This exploration, then, will be carried out in two phases – first, for the life cycle and then for the yearly one.

The word 'cycle' (although of Greek etymology) is in this context ours. Greek speaks rather of *hēlikiai* – 'ages' or 'life stages' – for the former sort of cycle, and *hōrai* – seasons – for the latter. The corresponding Latin words are, usually, *aetas* and *hora*. And, of course, not only are the units of division very different in each case – spans of years, on the one hand, and subdivisions of a single year, on the other – but there is a further, more fundamental distinction: that between a *single, linear* time-span, of variable length, on the one hand, and a series of *repeating, recurrent or revolving* time-spans, of fixed duration, on the other.[1]

Nonetheless, it makes sense to treat the two together. There is a close connection between them, in terms of both the physical theories involved and the relevance of these theories to everyday life, as well as to medical interventions and the understanding of medical conditions. Indeed, both the Greek *hōra* and the Latin *hora* in some cases *are* used also to refer to stages or times of life – another consideration which underscores the conceptual connection. Moreover, there are, as we shall see as we proceed, several texts which do explicitly draw the parallel between these two kinds of cycle, that of the seasons and that of the stages of life.[2]

---

[1] There is, undoubtedly, a conceptual connection to be made also between the cycle of seasons and the monthly cycle, or other cycles which take place within a month; both recurrence or periodicity, and astronomically or astrologically based phenomena and calculations, are central to both. In view of the highly technical nature of the latter kind of cycle, however, as it is understood in the medical discourse, and the distinct set of theoretical considerations that it raises, this has been treated separately, in chapter 4.

[2] E.g. 'Hippocrates', *Regimen* 3.2, coupling the age of the individual and the season of the year as factors which determine which exercises should be undertaken. We shall see such explicit

We shall consider the Graeco-Roman understanding of what happens to the human body in the course of these cycles. Such concepts as the fundamental qualities (e.g. the hot, the cold, the wet and the dry), the elements (e.g. earth, air, fire and water) and the fluids or humours (e.g. blood, phlegm, yellow bile and black bile) tend to be central in both cases. The different successive ages of the human being are understood in terms of a gradual progression from the predominance of one or more of these qualities or fluids to the predominance of others. The nature – and the medical significance and implications – of the different seasons, equally, are understood in terms of such successive or alternating dominations.

To be sure, there is nothing like universal agreement between medical authors – or between them and others – even within the classical Greek period, about these underlying constituents, or fundamental physiological processes, of the human body; nor, therefore, about the precise changes involved in the successive phases of either cycle – the life cycle or that of the seasons – or the appropriate medical interventions.[3] Within the medical texts, it will be informative to focus our attention mainly on texts of the 'Hippocratic corpus', which provide us with our most substantial evidence for the early, classical Greek period, and for the later period on those of Galen, which – as in many branches of ancient medical history – serve not just as outlets for his own medical views but as a major source for those of his predecessors and rivals.

The cycle of life: the ages of man (and woman) in the Graeco-Roman world

We may start with a fundamental distinction, between the understandings or perceptions of life phases and transitions which were obvious and central to

---

connections also in the 'Hippocratic' *Hebdomads* and in other medical texts discussed below; an analogical connection, between a country's young men and the spring of the year, is attributed to Pericles by Aristotle, *Rhetoric* 1.7, 1365a32 = 3.10, 1411a2; we may compare also Ovid, *Metamorphoses* 15.199–213, comparing the succeeding times of life to seasons of the year.

3 So, to give just a brief glimpse of the diversity, even within the so-called 'Hippocratic corpus', the text *Regimen* posits two constituent *elements* of the human body, fire and water, in contradistinction to the four *fluids* (blood, phlegm, yellow bile, black bile) of *The Nature of the Human Being*; other texts posit different selections of two or three fluids. For an overview of the varied texts of the corpus and their content, see Craik (2015); for a more radical caution, pointing to the arbitrary criteria of selection of the works in the corpus in its present form, and advocating the abandonment of the application to it of the term 'Hippocratic', even in quotation marks, see van der Eijk (2015a).

the conduct of life in the ancient world and the more theorized models through which medical authors and philosophers tried to 'rationalize' these.

Let us consider first the former. These will be closely dependent on observed changes in the human body, on the one hand, and on expectations of life roles and activities, on the other. At a broad level of understanding, we may think of the traditional perceptions of the nature of youth and of old age purveyed by such texts as Aristotle's *Rhetoric*, or by a range of Latin literary texts, such as those of Horace, Pliny the Younger, or Seneca.[4]

Taking a somewhat broader view, we may observe that archaic and classical Greek usage broadly reflects a four-age structure – child, youth, adult man, old man – albeit with some variations in the word used for each, which are closely tied to the social role or expectations in each case.[5] A similar pattern is found in Latin sources, with the succession childhood – youth (*adulescens/iuvenis*) – adult man – old man (*senex*).[6]

The perception of moments of transition will in many ways be more important than that of phases or spans of years, especially where the former are related to clear and dramatic rites of passage. Here – as indeed throughout this discourse regarding the life cycle – there is both a fundamental division between male and female, and a serious paucity of evidence in relation to the latter.

---

4 Aristotle (*Rhetoric* 2.12–14) presents youth and old age as two extremes, with excess and passion or strong emotion dominant in the former and the opposite characteristics, including lack of confidence and lack of generosity, in the latter, and the prime as a medial state free from either extreme. The psychological or moral changes are also, in the same way that we shall see in the medical texts, connected to an overall transition from heat to cold. In his *Art of Poetry* (156–78) Horace presents a four-stage picture: childhood (*puer*), youth (*iuvenis*), adulthood (*virilis*), old age (*senex*), with the standard behaviour and societal occupations associated with each. Seneca compares his own state in old age to that of a decaying house; we observed in the previous chapter the rather more positive account of the possible daily experience of old age suggested by Galen and Pliny the Younger.
5 As discussed by Falkner, the implied pattern in Homer is the succession: child (*pais*) – youth (*neos/kouros*) – man – old man (*gerōn / presbus*), and the structure related to the (male) person's military role, whereas similar divisions to be found in Hesiod are related rather to his potential for productive labour (e.g. *Works and Days* 131; 441–7; 695–7). *Neos* or *kouros* is the standard term for 'youth' in Homer and classical poetry, while *meirakion* or *neaniskos* tend to be later, or prose, words; the undifferentiated *anēr* ('man') in these earlier texts may correspond to the 'man in his prime', *akmazōn*, that we find in the philosophical and medical discourse; both *presbus* and *gerōn* are found in application to the last phase.
6 For the Roman life cycle and attitudes to the different life stages see Wiedemann (1989); Laurence (2000); Harlow and Laurence (2002); Cokayne (2003).

Indeed, the crucial transitional moment, that of marriage, is in some respects the only one that emerges as significant on the female side: it is difficult to extract from ancient literary sources any account of an overall female life cycle, or of its phases, beyond that provided by recommendations or accounts of the moment of marriage, which might typically take place at the age of 14 (or even earlier), and is obviously in some sense – albeit loosely – connected with the onset of puberty.[7]

An arguable exception to this paucity of sources on female life phases, however, is provided by the stereotype of the aged nurse or female attendant, for example in Epic and in Greek tragedy. Here we have a strongly age-specific type, namely that of a post-menopausal woman whose role is to perform domestic work and look after children in a higher-class household, but also to provide assistance and advice, sometimes of a gynaecologically specific nature. We also have evidence, especially in the contexts of midwifery and pharmacology, of women as practitioners and dispensers of traditional wisdom. It seems likely that the literary stereotype reflects a social reality which is related to our information from medical sources – that is to say, that it was women beyond childbearing age, in particular, who performed the roles of nurse, midwife and in some cases medical expert. To that extent, then, this does constitute a distinct life phase for some women, connected to their biological age. It is noteworthy that such a distinct 'late-life' phase is of applicability only to women of a lower social class, not to noblewomen or aristocrats.[8]

On the male side, however, we have much fuller evidence, regarding both moments of transition and successive life roles. In both classical Greek and classical Roman society, childhood was followed by a transitional stage, that of the *meirakion* or *neaniskos* in the former case and that of the *iuvenis* or *adulescens* in the latter, which involved – in the elite stratum of society which provides us with most of our evidence – a one- or two-year period of military service or military-

---

[7] On the poverty of evidence for female life stages see Laurence (2000), who points to the life of the Augustus' daughter Julia as the only 'case study' discussed in detail in the sources (see Suetonius, *Augustus* 63–4; *Tiberius* 7; Dio Cassius 54.8, 54.35, 57.18).

[8] I am grateful to Kassandra Miller for suggesting this perspective. Prominent literary examples of such older nurses or wise women are Eurycleia in Homer's *Odyssey* and the Nurse in Euripides' *Hippolytus*. On female medical practitioners see King (1998), ch. 9; Flemming (2000), (2007). (These were typically known as *maia* or *obstetrix*, though there is epigraphic evidence of women also classified as *iatros*, *iatrina* or *medica*.) There has been much scholarly discussion of the extent to which literary medical texts, e.g. those of the Hippocratic corpus, reflect a specifically female body of knowledge – especially as regards drugs – even though this knowledge is inevitably filtered by male authors. As well as the works just cited see Dean-Jones (1994); Totelin (2009).

style training, the *ephebate* in the former case and the *tirocinium* in the latter. In Roman society, transition from childhood to *adulescentia* was marked by a distinct ceremony, around the age of 14–16, involving the exchange of the coloured clothes of childhood, the *toga praetexta*, for the plain, adult *toga virilis*, alongside other rites of passage. In both Greek and Roman society, too, the transitional phase is associated with particular perceptions of sexual desirability, as well as possible expectations of sexual activity.[9] In the Roman context there is evidence of a further rite of passage, involving the first shaving of the beard, in later teenage years, while full adulthood – bringing with it both the possibility of marriage and the capacity to hold public office – arrives only at age 25.[10]

Much more detail could be given, both of the expectations and perceptions surrounding these rites of passage, as evidenced in literary and epigraphic sources, and about the precise differences between the Roman and the Greek context, and indeed different Greek contexts, on both a geographical and a chronological basis. That would take us far beyond our present scope. The fundamental point should be noted, however, that the establishment of the chronological *moment* of these crucial transitions or phases is based either on the completion of a fixed number of years, or on observed physical changes, or on some combination of the two. For example, it seems that entry to the ephebate in archaic and classical Greek cities was tied to particular chronological age, around 18. On the one hand, this was later than the moment of transition to *adulescentia* for the Roman male; on the other hand, there seems to have been flexibility in the latter case, the child's father or guardian deciding the precise moment at which he would undergo the ceremony, presumably at least partially on the basis of an assessment of his perceived physical readiness.

The transition to full adulthood, meanwhile, at least to the extent that it is understood in terms of legal capacities and responsibilities, will be tied to a fixed chronological age; while that to old age, on the other hand – as we shall see fur-

---

9 There is a large literature on sexuality and permitted or expected sexual roles as related to different ages in the ancient world, where male adulthood emerges as the demarcator of active, as distinct from passive, sexual activity. See the classic works of Dover (1978/1989); Halperin (1990); Halperin, Winkler and Zeitlin (1990); Winkler (1991); and on the Roman context Walters (1997). More recently, Davidson (2001, 2007) has offered a more nuanced view of the dynamics of Graeco-Roman erotic relationships, undermining the simplistic statement of the nature of the active–passive distinction, as well as the over-emphasis on penetrative acts, that had dominated much late twentieth-century scholarship. But the fundamental point remains that there is a particular focus on a distinct, transitional phase of youth (*ephēbos, meirakion, neaniskos, iuvenis*) as both developmentally crucial and, in some contexts, uniquely desirable.
10 See Laurence (2000), citing Dio Cassius 52.20, as well as the *lex plaetoria* and *lex villia annalis*.

ther when we look in more detail at the medical discussions – was much more fluid, in terms of the determination of an actual number of years.

It should be noted, however, that in literary texts the age categories and periods so far considered appear almost always without any mention of numbers of years. Connections with precise ages come either from such legal stipulations as those just mentioned or from the more technical texts which we shall now proceed to explore.

Let us turn then to the other side of the distinction with which we started, that is, to the theorized models and rationalizations of the 'ages of man' that are given in various medical and other ancient discussions. Alongside the notion of rationalization, here, we should consider another, that of quantification, or the ambition to attach precise number of years to each life stage – although it should be clarified that the two projects – that of theorization, or rationalization, and that of applying precise numbers – do not always go hand in hand. Medical texts, for example, which give physiologically based accounts of the different ages do not always tie the changes in question to exact periods of years. (And, conversely, there is – as indeed we have just seen – *some* degree of arithmetical precision in the traditional understanding of life phases, too.)

But the attempt to arrive at precise numbers for the successive life phases is, to some extent, a recurrent preoccupation – and, we may say, a recurrent problem – of our sources. We shall see, too, that such numerical precision is more prominent, and *less* problematic, for the earlier phases than for the later ones. This, we may think, is understandable enough: for us, too, and in a way which at least to some degree transcends chronological and geographical diversity, earlier life developments – e. g. the appearance of teeth, cognitive changes, biological changes associated with puberty – may be clearly observed and tied to particular ages, while a division of the latter phases of life into equally neat chronological units will encounter the inconvenience, not just of widely diverging individual experiences of physical and cognitive decline, but also, not least, of age at death.

Some qualifications should doubtless be made to that observation. There are – again, for us too – *some* fixed, or relatively precise, markers of significance in the later phases of life too, provided either by biological reality (or the perception of it) or by societal convention, or by a combination of the two. One may think here of the strict designation of 'geriatric pregnancy' for pregnancies experienced over the age of 35, on the one hand, or of fixed retirement ages of 60 or 65, on the other; and one could add other examples of medical protocols related to particular older age groups – the recommendation of certain regular tests over the age of 50, for example. It seems overwhelmingly the case, however, that precise as opposed to more fluid age periods and markers will be of more relevance to earlier and formative ages than to later ones.

A stricture made by Aristotle in this context – one which we may, indeed, think sensible in its own right – is relevant to such ancient attempts, to which we now turn, to fix the stage of life in terms of precise periods of years. 'The discussion of those who divide the stages of life (*hēlikiai*) into seven-year periods (*hebodmades*) is in general terms not a bad one; but one must follow the division actually presented by nature (*phusis*).'[11]

For one form that the preoccupation with numerical exactitude takes is the project of dividing the human life span into seven-year periods (*hebdomades*), the number itself having powerful connotations, and the division into seven many other applications – enduring connotations and applications which in some ways have survived even into the modern world.[12] Both a poem attributed to the sixth-century lawgiver Solon and a 'Hippocratic' medical text, *Hebdomads*, present us with a clear and neat division into such seven-year periods, although the former text offers ten such periods and the latter seven.[13]

---

11 *Politics* 7.17, 1336b40–1337a1 (οἱ γὰρ τοῖς ἑβδομάσι διαιροῦντες τὰς ἡλικίας ὡς ἐπὶ τὸ πολὺ λέγουσιν οὐ κακῶς, δεῖ δὲ τῇ διαιρέσει τῆς φύσεως ἐπακολουθεῖν). In the rest of the discussion in the *Politics*, as well as elsewhere, Aristotle works broadly within the framework of a distinction into youth, prime and old age.

12 The importance of the number seven could be explored, from an anthropological or psychological perspective, in ways which would take us far beyond the present discussion. I confine myself to noting the conceptual importance of the seven-year cycle in the ancient biblical and related contexts, on which see e.g. Carmichael (1999); Casperson (2003); Krinis (2016), and in modern psychology the number seven was thought, and with some reservations may still be thought, to have a particular significance, as representing a natural limit to our information-processing ability; see Miller (1956), with Baddeley (1994). I am grateful to Yadin Dudai for drawing my attention to the latter literature. The division of the human lifespan into seven-year periods, for educational or developmental purposes, still retains its attraction, at least at the level of popular psychology, and is a well-known feature for example of the educational theory and practice of the Rudolf Steiner schools.

13 The most common sense of the term *hebdomas* came to be – as with its cognate in modern Greek – that of 'week', and this is so also in Galen, as we shall see in chapter 4. The project of the 'Hippocratic' *Hebdomads* is indeed precisely that of detecting the number 7 in as many human and cosmological contexts as possible – planets, winds, seasons, etc. Both a relationship with Pythagoreanism and an influence from astrology have been suggested (see e.g. Roscher 1906). It is noteworthy however that a quite different division is explicitly attributed to Pythagoras, by Diogenes Laertius (8.10), that of four life stages, each of twenty years' duration (though the division seems suspect, not just in terms of its viability in relation to lived experience, but perhaps also in terms of its likelihood to have been advanced by a Greek speaker, with the category of child covering the first twenty years, and 'young man' covering the ages of 40 to 60).

Solon's text has been read as a conscious polemic against ancient perceptions, especially those concerning old age;[14] whatever the truth of that, its highly theoretical division arguably takes us still further from Aristotle's 'following of nature' – or even from traditional Greek categories – than that of the Hippocratic text. The latter offers us the following succession: *paidion, pais, meirakion, neēniskos, anēr, presbutēs* and *gerōn*.

As already observed, the project of offering a definite numerical span for either adulthood itself or the phases of old age is one which encounters very obvious problems – problems which in fact receive different attempted solutions both within this text itself and in its subsequent tradition. First, the text itself does not, in fact, offer a straightforward picture of seven sevens. As if in acknowledgement of the problem we have noted, two deviations are made from the scheme, the core adult phase *anēr* being allotted two *hebdomades* rather than one, and the final phase of *gerōn* not being set any fixed limit. (See table 1.)

TABLE 1: Ages in the 'Hippocratic' *Hebdomads*

Life stage	Numerical age
paidion	to age 7
pais	to age 14
meirakion	to age 21
neēniksos	to age 28
anēr	to age 49
presbutēs	to age 56
gerōn	56 onward

We might say that the text thus allows two departures from the artificiality of its model in the direction of lived reality. A couple of later authors who refer to this text handle the problem in slightly different ways, in one case insisting on fixed time periods for the last two ages, but extending both of them, so that the life of a *presbutēs* extends to the end of the ninth hebdomad (age 63) and that of the *gerōn* from there to the end of the fourteenth (age 98), in other cases making other adjustments.[15]

---

14 See Falkner (1990).
15 See West (1971): 376.

The strict division of the latter phases of life on the basis of any set of fixed periods, then, is undoubtedly problematic. The same procedure as applied to the first four *hebdomades*, meanwhile – the first twenty-eight years of life – may be rather more promising. As we shall see shortly in the work of Galen, and other medical authors, the division of the earlier phases of life into these segments was indeed taken as having genuine significance, in terms of biological development and of the appropriate health care and education at each phase. The connection of the age of 14 with pubertal change is clearly central to this;[16] but a further division of childhood into a first and a second *hebdomas*, as well as an understanding of full adulthood or maturity as reached only at 28 – and possibly also of age 35 as the beginning of a decline – will also emerge as features which are tied to genuine perceived transitions.

Medical authors on the life stages

We turn our attention, then, to physiological and medical discussions. Central to these is the notion of the successive dominance of a different element or quality in the body at the different stages of life. More broadly, the conception whereby the perceptible qualities or stuffs in the human body are essentially the same as, or composed of, a small number of fundamental elements or qualities that also compose the external universe seems present in, or at least implied by, a range of Presocratic physical theories; this is seen clearly, at least, in Empedocles of Acragas.[17] It seems likely, too, that the view that there are different levels of heat or moisture at different stages of life – in particular the association of hotness with youth, or of coldness with old age – reflects widely-held traditional perceptions. Plato associates infancy with moisture, and childhood and youth with heat, in a way which is related to his own four-element theory. Aristotle, too, coordinates the behavioural development from youth, through the prime, to old age with a

---

16 On this see Aristotle, *Historia Animalium* 5.14, 544b23–8, associating pubertal change with *hēbē*, and mentioning 14 as the age at which seed is first produced (though he does not think it fertile until 21); cf. *Politics* 7.17, 1336b37–40, where the watershed of *hēbē*, occurring roughly though not precisely at age 14, seems to correspond to puberty. On this point see further below on Galen, where the significance of sexual change as an age demarcator seems at best hinted at, rather than clearly present. See also Eyben (1972); Kleijwegt (1991).

17 For Empedocles the four fundamental elements, or 'roots', in the cosmos (fire, earth, air and water) also function in the account of how humans come into being (see Empedocles A21, A30, A49, B6, B23 and B27 DK); moreover it is by these elements within the body that we perceive those without (B84, B109 DK), and the differential mixture of elements in the blood is responsible for differences in character (B86 DK).

diminution in heat; and he also conceives the aging process, on an analogy with that of plants, as a gradual drying out of the body.[18]

Neither in these philosophical texts nor in the classical medical ones, however, does any such clear or neat division of stages of life appear as those considered above, and certainly none which attempts to tie such stages to numerical spans of years.[19]

The closest thing we find to such a neat scheme in the 'Hippocratic' texts is perhaps the discussion in *Regimen* (1.33, 150 Joly/Byl, VI.510–12 L.), linking each of the four traditional stages of life with a pairing of the four fundamental qualities, hot, cold, wet and dry. The picture that emerges from that chapter is that given in Table 2.

TABLE 2: A standard 'Hippocratic' age division (from *Regimen* 1.33)

Life stage	Physical qualities
Child (*pais*)	wet and hot
Youth (*neēniskos*)	dry and hot
Adult man (*anēr*)	dry and cold
Old man (*gerōn*)	wet and cold

Elsewhere in the classical Greek medical texts, such classificatory detail about the stages of life is hard to find, nor is the above scheme necessarily followed precisely. A similar scheme, however, but with further subdivision and further detail regarding changes around puberty, is implied by a text from the Hippocrat-

---

18 Plato, as cited by Galen, links infancy with excessive moisture: *Timaeus* 43a6–8, 43b5–c1, 44a8–b9, quoted and discussed at *The Soul's Dependence on the Body* 4, 42–4 Müller (IV.780–2 K.). Even if Galen's physicalist interpretation here is over-literal, Plato's overall view seems to be one where youth is hot, and where there is a gradual diminution of moisture – or hardening – in old age. See *Laws* 2, 666a3–c2, which makes both these points, with the analogy for the drinking of wine by minors of 'driving fire upon fire', and the characterization of old age by contrast as hard and in need of softening (and therefore of wine). For Aristotle's association of different ages with different levels of heat, see again *Rhetoric* 2.12–14; for old age as a withering or drying out, *Respiration* 17, 478b27–8.

19 As touched on already, Aristotle suggests an *approximate* use of the notion of seven-year periods (nn. 11, 16), though he also mentions earlier ages, such as 5, as watersheds for educational or nurturing purposes (*Politics* 7.17, 1336a23). He also gives an approximate age of 30–35 for the prime of the body and 49 for that of the soul: *Rhetoric* 2.14, 1390b9–11; cf. *Politics* 7.17, 1335b29–37, placing the peak of intelligence around age 50, and mentioning a point four or five years after that as a limit after which people should refrain from reproducing.

ic *Aphorisms* (3.24–31, 130–2 Loeb, IV.496–502 L.). The passage individuates the following stages of life as prone to different pathologies (examples of which are given in parentheses in each case): newborn or small children (vomiting, coughing, insomnia, fears); period of teething (gum irritation, fever, convulsions); older children (inflammation of the tonsils, asthma, stone, worms); still older children, approaching maturity (*hēbē*) (the same, plus longer-lasting fevers and nosebleeds); young men (acute fevers, epilepsy); men older than that (pleurisy, pneumonia, lethargy, phrenitis, burning fever, diarrhoea, haemorrhoids); old men (difficulty in breathing, joint pains, kidney complaints, apoplexy, insomnia, watery discharges). It is noteworthy here, too, in relation to our consideration above of crucial transitional moments in life, that the period of *hēbē*, in both boys and girls, receives particular attention: 'those children's diseases that persist and do not cease at the *hēbē*, or in girls at the onset of menstruation, usually become chronic'.

Undoubtedly the most striking association between a particular disease and a transitional time of life, however, is that presented in the Hippocratic text *Diseases of Girls*, in relation to the menarche. More generally in the gynaecological Hippocratic texts, there is a focus on the presence of menstruation in the absence of marriage or sexual activity – especially, for example in the case of women recently widowed – as potentially dangerous and pathological. It is in this context especially that we encounter the famous 'hysteria' or 'hysterical suffocation' (i.e., suffocation of the womb). In this text, more dramatically, a particular syndrome is identified as afflicting girls at the onset of puberty – a syndrome that involves a variety of disturbed and deranged behaviour, sometimes leading even to suicide.[20]

Leaving aside such specific, acute pathologies associated with this particular transitional stage, however – and while it is important not to overstate the coherence or univocal nature of these classical Greek medical texts – we may say in very broad terms that a picture emerges whereby heat tends to predominate at an earlier stage, and cold (and, according to some, moisture) at a later stage, with related pathologies. And of course, diet and medical interventions will reflect this.

---

[20] The relevant texts, and the conception of the female body implied by them, are fully explored by Dean-Jones (1994); King (1998). The adolescent syndrome identified by *Diseases of Girls* has been most recently discussed by Totelin (2021), who focuses on its connection with water and the perceived fluidity of the female body.

Thus, in a less differentiated way than that implied by the above four-stage model, book 1 of the *Epidemics* distinguishes – within the context of an epidemic outbreak – between certain conditions predominantly affecting children, others affecting women and others 'those who were older (*presbuteroisi*), in whom the hot is already mastered' (62, II.638 L.).[21]

Let us turn to Galen, our main source for the later, Roman imperial, period. In his account of the stages of human life, as in so many other areas, Galen claims to follow 'Hippocrates', while in fact adding a lot of detail not to be found in Hippocratic texts, which indeed from the point of view of his analysis would seem to conflate certain important categories. (It should be noted here that the 'Hippocratic' text we considered above, *Hebdomads*, is not amongst those which Galen considers authentic or follows in his views.[22]) In the process, I will suggest, Galen offers two particularly interesting contributions to our understanding of ancient attitudes to different times of life and the education or care relevant to them.

Now, Galen nowhere lays out his views on the successive phases or times of life with complete clarity; there is no text devoted specially to that theme. However, a fairly clear picture emerges, albeit with some variations in detail. There are either four or five main stages: childhood, prime, post-prime and old age, or the same, with the insertion of youth or adolescence between childhood and the prime. There is a close connection between these phases and the *hebdomades* that we have already encountered, although – again as previously suggested – these *hebdomades* are clearly of more relevance to earlier than to later stages.

The physical theory underpinning the scheme, meanwhile, is that of the composition of our bodies from four fundamental qualities – the hot, the cold, the wet and the dry. For Galen, aging consists in a gradual diminution in both heat and moisture; however, heat remains largely constant from infancy to the end of the prime, at least in optimal cases, while moisture begins to diminish

---

[21] Later in the same passage three different categories of youth or young adult are lumped together as having been more likely to die: *neoi*, *meirakia* and *akmazontes* (though this does not admittedly mean that the author makes no conceptual distinction between these).

[22] The textual history is slightly complicated here. Galen is aware of and refers to a text 'on hebdomads' (although this is only part of the text that has come down to us under that title – the part, indeed, which focusses on divisions into 7 parts); and he refers to this as a work 'attributed to Hippocrates', e. g. *Commentary on Hippocrates' Epidemics, book 1* 1.1, 13 Wenkebach and Pfaff (XVIIA.18 K.), where his comment is on what is said about *seasons*. The work in the form that we have it is however referred to and extensively commented on by a pseudo-Galenic author of a period close to Galen's.

from infancy onwards. This view of the constancy of heat in the earlier stages of life represents a bone of contention between Galen and other theorists, as does another theoretical point on which he insists: the fact that old people's bodies are drier, not wetter, than at the prime be obscured by the greater build-up of fluids, such as phlegm, within those bodies. That is: old people are indeed drier, in terms of their solid bodies, but they may accumulate a deceptive quantity of fluids – mucus, phlegm – within or between those solid bodies. This leads to a confusion on the part of some of Galen's rivals, who falsely characterize old age as wet. (As we have seen above, in doing so they follow a model which in fact has solid Hippocratic justification, in the text *Regimen*.)[23]

It is thus the case for Galen that – as we also saw also in the discussion presented by the Hippocratic *Aphorisms*, above – certain diseases are more typically associated with certain ages. 'Cold' diseases in general are those of old age, as 'hot' ones of youth.[24] There are age-based differences in the prevalence of acute diseases, too: discussion of a Hippocratic text which speaks of those under 30 being more prone to abscesses, those of 30 above rather to quartan fevers, leads Galen to elaborate on such distinctions.[25]

In accordance with the hebdomadal division which holds, as we have seen, at least for the first phases, certain kinds of lifestyle practice and habituation are recommended during the first seven-year period, which are continued in largely the same way up to the age of fourteen, with the addition of certain kinds of ethical and intellectual education.[26] These two seven-year periods together constitute childhood. (A further subdivision may be added, as the category of *brephos*, infant, is sometimes discussed separately from that of the child, *pais*.)[27] Fourteen is – as again we have observed in other discussions – a pivotal age; and it is here that we encounter what seems to me the first of Galen's particularly illuminating contributions to the ancient discourse on age. From this point, he says, over the third seven-year period, the training and education of different persons may di-

---

23 See *Health* 1.12, 28,15–21 Koch (VI.59–60 K.); and, more polemically, *Mixtures* 2.2, where the proponents of the alternative views (childhood as hotter than the prime, and old age as wet) are not mentioned by name, but seem to be numerous and perhaps represent the majority view. As we have seen (nn. 4 and 18 above), both Plato's and Aristotle's developmental view certainly involve a diminution of heat between childhood or youth and adulthood, though they seem to be in agreement with Galen on the dry quality of old age.
24 See e.g. *Mixtures* 2.6, 46 Helmreich (I.582 K.), giving a list of 'cold diseases' to which the old are prone: 'apoplexy, paralysis, numbness, tremor, convulsion, mucus, sore throats'.
25 *Critical Days* 3.11 (IX.754–8 K.).
26 *Health* 1.12, 28,12–31 Koch (VI.59–60 K.).
27 See again *Mixtures* 2.2, and note the dedicated discussion of the earliest stage of nurture at *Health* 1.7–10.

verge quite radically, depending on the individual character and expected role in life.

> if you wish to bring him to the peak of good-condition – say you want to make him a noble soldier, a wrestler, or some other kind of strong person – you will take less care of the goods of the soul, at least of those goods which lead towards some kind of scientific knowledge and wisdom; for matters concerning character should be addressed with precision at this stage of life especially. If, on the other hand, you choose to limit bodily matters to the strengthening of the parts, the acquisition of some sort of healthy condition, and growth, while your major concern is the improvement of the youth's soul – you will not require the same daily regime in both cases. And indeed a third and a fourth form of lifestyle may be found: that of those who engage in some manual specialized skill – which in turn may either involve the body in physical exercise or leave it unexercised – and that of those who engage in farming or business or some other such thing. So it actually seems quite difficult to enumerate all the types of life.[28]

We have here an acknowledgement of different patterns or models of life, and of different patterns of early education and training appropriate to each, which is remarkable, if not unique, within the medical and philosophical discourses.

The age of fourteen, or in some cases a little later, also corresponds to the beginning of the phase Galen calls *hēbaskein* – which could be translated as 'to be youthful' or perhaps 'to reach maturity'. An obvious translation might be 'puberty', although it is rather striking that while other texts mention sexual development as a key feature at this age, Galen does not seem to be explicit about the connection between the age of 14 and sexual development – except to the extent that such development may be taken as connoted by the term *hēbaskein* itself. Nor, indeed, does he focus on sexual development as central to changes in health care or lifestyle.[29]

It is, however, important to bear in mind, throughout all this, that Galen explicitly states that precise numbers cannot be put on the life phases under discussion.[30]

The period from fourteen to twenty-one would seem to be, or certainly to include, that of the *ephēbos* ('adolescent') and the *meirakion* ('youth'). It seems either that the prime proper begins after that, or that the *ephēbos–meirakion* stage

---

[28] *Health* 1.12, 28,32–29,8 Koch (VI.60–1 K.). Again, Aristotle's identification of the stages of 7 to *hēbē* and *hēbē* to 20 as crucial to education (see nn. 16, 19 above) clearly represents some relevant background to this.
[29] By contrast, we note that pubertal change – the beginning of seed production – is a crucial medical demarcator in Soranus, at least as far as women are concerned (*Gynaecology* 1.20).
[30] See *Health* 6.2, 170,32–35 Koch (VI.387 K.), both for this caveat and for the mention of *hēbaskein*.

(which is not in fact mentioned in most of Galen's summaries of the phases of life)[31] itself constitutes the beginning of the 'prime'. Where the transitional stage *is* mentioned, it is stated to be that of best mixture – although perhaps not in a way which significantly distinguishes it from the prime more generally[32] – and certainly Galen, from his medical perspective, evinces none of the interest in the *social* significance of the *ephēbos–meirakion* stage as a rite of passage which we observed above.

He does, however, state explicitly that the 'post-prime' begins in some cases at 30, in others as late as 35. It is tempting to try to tie the beginning of the 'post-prime' very approximately to the conclusion of the fourth seven-year period, and incidentally Galen does mention the age of 28 as in a sense pivotal in his own development. Whether by coincidence of not, it turned out to be a crucial turning-point in his own life.

> Yet during my childhood, and even my adolescence (*ephēbos*) and youth (*meirakion*) I fell victim to quite a large number of sicknesses. It was after the completion of my twenty-eighth year that I became convinced that there was such a thing as the art of health and took to following its injunctions; and I have continued to do so throughout my subsequent life, with the result that I never suffered any disease other than a very occasional ephemeral fever. These too, of course, can be avoided by those who choose a life free of obligations, as has become clear in what was said previously ...[33]

---

31 Galen suffered from certain illnesses as a child, a *meirakion* and *ephēbos*; see *Health* 5.1, 136,27–32 Koch (VI.309 K.), where he contrasts this phase as a whole with his experience after the age of 28. At *Health* 6.2, 171,1–2 Koch (VI.387 K.), he moves from the mention of *hēbaskein* straight on to the *post*-prime, beginning around 30 or 35, again perhaps implying that the former, around age 14, is indeed the beginning of the prime. In the *Commentary on Hippocrates' Nature of the Human Being* Galen gives the fourfold, rather than the fivefold, division: childhood, prime, post-prime, old age (3.7, 94,26–95,1 Mewaldt, XV.186 K.), again without precise ages.
32 'The best mixture of the body is that which it possesses at the time of youth (*meirakia*), while all others are inferior to this', *Health* 6.2, 170,28–9 Koch. (VI.387 K.); 'the time between that of children and those in their prime, which is that of *ephēboi* and *meirakia*, should be that with the best mixture', *Commentary on Hippocrates' Nature of the Human Being* 3.7, 95,11–13 Mewaldt (XV.187 K.). *Meirakia* and people in their prime are classed together in terms of their heat at *Commentary on Hippocrates' Epidemics, book 1*. 1.12, 31,28–30 Wenkebach (XVIIA.54 K.); cf. ibid. 2.80, 92–5 Wenkebach (XVIIA.183–187 K.). At *Commentary on Hippocrates Epidemics, book 6*, 3.28, 165,20–24 Wenkebach (XVIIB.77 K.), the stage of *ephēboi* and *meirakia* is transitional between those of child and man, and such changes are gradual rather than sudden. But at least one specific age corresponding to *meirakion* is given: at *The Therapeutic Method* 5.12 (X.366 K.) and *The Therapeutic Method to Glaucon* 1.9 (XI.28 K.) an eighteen-year-old is described with that term.
33 *Health* 5.1, 136 Koch (VI.309 K.).

Be that as it may, what is clear is that post-prime corresponds to a loss of vigour, connected to the gradual loss of moisture and heat which characterizes the aging process, and that these losses become still more marked as one proceeds into old age itself. It seems, also, that the numerical age at which one first becomes old (*gerōn*) is even less clearly demarcated than that of the onset of the post-prime – a reasonable acknowledgement on Galen's part, one may think, of the individual variations in speed of the aging process.

Intriguingly – and perhaps uniquely in the literature – Galen offers a further subtlety, regarding the progress of old age. He individuates three further stages, which correspond to different levels of feebleness and of coldness: 'fresh', 'wrinkled' and 'proceeding' old age.[34]

It should be mentioned, finally, that while the progress from childhood, and in particular from the prime, to old age, is seen as one of a gradual loss of vigour, Galen asserts a difference here between the quality of physical or natural (*phusikai*) and that of 'soul' or mental (*psuchikai*) activities: the former are at their best in childhood, the latter after childhood up to the post-prime.[35]

Table 3 represents an attempted reconstruction of the Galenic picture of the different stages of life – albeit a somewhat tentative one, given the uncertainties and fluidities already identified.

TABLE 3: The stages of life in Galen

Main life stage	Further or subsidiary life stage	Numerical age
Childhood (*Pais*)		0–7 and 7–14
	Infancy (*brephos*)	0–2
Prime (*Akmazōn*)		21 (or 14?)–c.30/35
	Ephēbos / Meirakion	c. 14–21 (?)
Post-Prime (*Parakmazōn*)		c.30/35–?
Old Age (*Gerōn*)		?–?
	Fresh Old Age (*Ōmogerōn*)	
	Middle Old Age (*Suphar*)	
	Extreme Old Age (*Pempelos*)	

---

34 *Health* 5.12, 167,17–19 Koch (VI.379–80 K.). The latter two terms are highly unusual in Greek, and the last indeed represents a disputed reading of the text; see Singer's (forthcoming) note at loc.
35 *Health* 6.2, 170,30–32 Koch (VI.387 K.). By *psuchikos* in this context Galen clearly seems to mean mental or intellectual capacities.

It is in Galen's discussion of old age and its care, however, especially in his major work on healthy regimen or preventive medicine, *Health*, that we encounter another of his most interesting perspective on times of life, their conceptualization and treatment. For, in spite of the overall picture of gradual decline from the age of 35 or so which his model entails, Galen is in fact strikingly optimistic about the possibility of the maintenance of health, even to an advanced old age. Provided two conditions hold, such prolonged good health should be perfectly achievable.

The first of these conditions consists in careful attention to the precepts of healthy living, as laid out by Galen in his treatise. Here what is crucial above all is to understand the nature of the individual constitution, and to try to maintain it in its current state, not introducing any major or unexpected alterations, but at the same time to be aware of pathological departures – for example those that arise from the excessive build-up of one or other fluid – and address these promptly.

The second condition is the good fortune not to be afflicted by a disease 'from outside' as opposed to one arising from within the body. Though the terminology seems unspecific, what is being acknowledged here is the existence of such unpredictable external events as outbreaks of epidemic disease or indeed plague (something that Galen has himself lived through for considerable periods), or of bodily injuries, all of which may have serious, even fatal, consequences, however careful one is with one's daily regime.[36] In the absence of these, however, one should be able to prolong life, and prolong it in health, for many years. This is made clear by the quotation we just considered, as well as by the two examples of health in old age, those of Antiochus and Telephus, which we considered in a different context in the previous chapter.

The yearly cycle: the seasons

In the case of the seasons of year, again, what is central is the notion of a succession or alternation of predominant physical qualities, with attendant conse-

---

36 See *Health* 5.1, 136 Koch (VI.308 K.). Although there was no clear conception of contagion or infectious disease at the period in question (on the history of which concept see Nutton (1983), who however perhaps overstates the limited extent to which such a concept *can* be identified in Galen), plague or infectious disease must surely be amongst the 'external' or 'from outside' diseases – those which cannot be predicted or kept in check simply by diet and daily regime. (Galen will talk, though not of air-borne disease, of 'ambient air' as a crucial factor in this context.)

quences in terms of the most frequent pathologies, as well as the appropriate lifestyle prescriptions or medical interventions, in each case.

Before we come to these, let us give a brief outline of the main Graeco-Roman divisions of the year. Although we will concentrate on discussions from medical texts in what follows, the divisions of the year which they present, tied as they are to the observation of a combination of seasonal changes and astronomical phenomena, are fundamentally the same as, or a more nuanced development of, those we find already in archaic texts.[37]

It will by this stage not be surprising to find out that there were those who were keen to individuate seven seasons in the year. Such a division is given by our now familiar *Hebdomads* text. It does, however, seem to have some solid basis and validity beyond that theoretical text: the seven-part division was related to the different agricultural activities undertaken throughout the year, and such a variant on the simpler four-part division is acknowledged also by Galen in his commentary on the first book of the Hippocratic *Epidemics*.[38] However, as both Hippocratic and Galenic discussions agree – and as supported by other classical texts – the general consensus is that there are four seasons, even if there may be some significant subdivisions or other crucial moments within them. These four, with the points of division between them, are outlined in the Hippocratic *Regimen*,[39] as summarized in the Table 4. (The same text in fact does present further subdivisions of the main four seasons, as we shall see shortly.)

We should pause here to clarify the ancient understanding of the motions of the heavenly bodies, which provides the backdrop against which these observations and seasonal divisions are to be understood.

The ancient model of the heavens – which corresponds to the observed situation from earth – is based on the understanding that we are located on the surface of one sphere (the earth) and looking outwards at the inside of another sphere, that of the heavens, to which the stars are fixed. (See figure 7.) This whole celestial sphere of the fixed stars rotates around the earth, the stars appearing to

---

[37] For further detail see Hannah (2005), especially chapters 1 and 2 on the early Greek developments; the main essential markers of the seasons which we shall consider in more detail below appear already in some form in Homer and even more so in Hesiod, where they are tied to agricultural activities.

[38] Our now familiar *Hebdomads* gives *sporatos* ('sowing'), winter, *phutaliai* ('planting'), spring, summer, autumn and late-autumn (*metopōron*), thus dividing winter into three parts and also adding a further division within autumn. Galen acknowledges a similar seven-part division at *Commentary on Hippocrates Epidemics, book 1* 1.1, 13 Wenkebach and Pfaff (XVIIA.18 K.).

[39] 3.68, 194–200 Joly/Byl (VI.594–604 L.).

move from east to west, and completes one revolution in approximately one day. The sun rotates around us too, in the same direction, but at a slightly slower speed.

TABLE 4: Divisions of the seasons (according to *Regimen*)

Season	Starting point	End point	Duration
winter (*cheimōn*)	heliacal setting of Pleiades [end of October]	spring equinox	144 days
spring (*ear*)	spring equinox	heliacal rising of Pleiades [mid-May]	54 days
summer (*theros*)	heliacal rising of Pleiades [mid-May]	heliacal rising of Arcturus [mid-September]	122 days
autumn (*phthino-pōron*)	heliacal rising of Arcturus [mid-September]	heliacal setting of Pleiades [late October]	45 days

Because of the slight discrepancy in speeds, the sun appears gradually to slip back in the sky each day in relation to the other stars; that is to say, different stars or constellations are observed just before sunrise or just after sunset in the course of the year, so that the sun may be said to be 'in' these different constellations at those different dates.

This observed path of the sun's motion in relation to the sphere of the fixed stars over the course of the year is known as the ecliptic. (The ecliptic describes a circle around the earth tilted at an angle of 23.5 degrees with respect to the celestial equator – that is, the line of the equator extended outwards onto that fixed sphere of the stars.) The zodiac can be thought of as a broad band drawn on the circumference of the fixed celestial sphere, following the line of the ecliptic, and with the twelve zodiac signs or constellations spaced equally along it. Because of the above 'slippage', then, the sun is perceived to proceed along his band in the course of the year. How far it has proceeded – its position in the zodiac – can be ascertained by the observation of which constellation appears just after the sun has set, and in the place where it has set on the horizon. So, the 'progress' of the sun through the zodiac is actually the phenomenon that – again, from our viewpoint on earth – the fixed sphere rotates somewhat faster than the sun, so that each month the sun slips back to an earlier point – a different zodiac sign – along the band.

The 'planets' – which on the ancient understanding include the sun and the moon – derive their name (*planētai* = 'wanderers') precisely from the fact that their motion is not the same as that of the sphere of the fixed stars: they com-

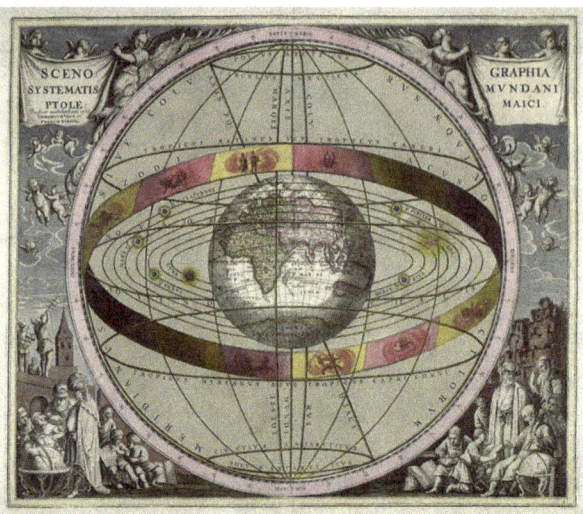

Figure 7: The two-sphere model of the cosmos, showing the fixed outer sphere of the stars, with the band of the zodiac marked upon it. Also shown are the separate motions of the 'planets'. From Andreas Cellarius, *Harmonia macrocosmica*, 1708, depiction of the Ptolemaeic view. Source: https://commons.wikimedia.org/wiki/Category:Cellarius_Harmonia_Macrocosmica#/media/File:Cellarius_Harmonia_macrocosica_1708_Scenographia_systematis_mundani_ptolemaici.jpg

plete their revolutions around the earth at different speeds. The other planets too, including the moon, are to be observed at different points on (or very near) the ecliptic, and thus can also be understood as interacting with the zodiac.

The 'heliacal rising' or 'heliacal setting' of stars or constellations is, similarly, a function of the difference in speed between the two revolutions. Here, 'rising' refers to the first moment in the year at which the constellation becomes visible in the sky just before dawn, after a period of invisibility, 'setting' to the last point in the year at which it is visible in the evening just before sunset, before its return to that period of invisibility. In the course of the year, different stars and constellations are observed in the night sky just before dawn (heliacal rising) or just before sunset (heliacal setting). (See figure 8.)

Thus, as is evident from the above table, the heliacal rising and setting of certain constellations were traditionally accepted dividing points of the year. The text in question in fact uses several such dividing points, in combination with those provided by the equinoxes. The result is a very uneven division of

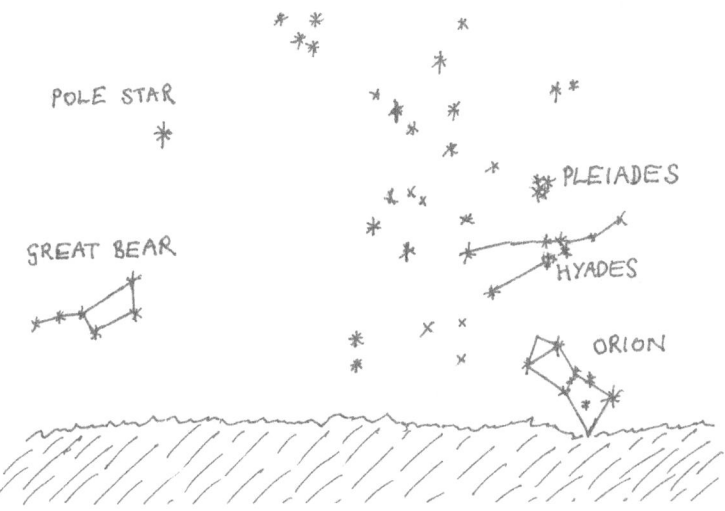

Figure 8: The heliacal rising of the Pleiades, Hyades and Orion. The drawing shows the sky as observed just before dawn at the beginning of summer from a location in mainland Greece: the first visibility of certain stars and constellations at this time functioned as indicators of the transitions between seasons. After Hannah (2009), 23.

the year, for which there is doubtless a traditional, agricultural basis, wherein most of the spring and autumn are subsumed into summer and winter.[40]

As suggested previously, there is a significant connection, in medical terms, between this meteorological or cosmic cycle of the seasons and that already discussed, of the stages of life. The connection is in fact made clear right from the outset in one of the best-known and most influential of classical Greek medical texts, the Hippocratic *Epidemics*. The text begins with an account of the climatic

---

40 The point is made by Hannah (2009: 47), on whom I have relied for the dates given in square brackets in the table and for the estimates of durations in days given in the last column. Further points of importance – also from an agricultural point of view – throughout the year were also identified, and were marked sequentially by the placement of pegs on physical calendars, known as *parapēgmata*, of which we have archaeological remains; see the comprehensive account of Lehoux (2007).

conditions at particular seasons of the year in one particular place, and of pestilential symptoms which arose in that context. It follows the progress of these climatic conditions from autumn through winter and spring to summer,[41] and in close conjunction also discusses the effects of the pestilence on a particular age range ('this happened to lads (*meirakia*), young men (*neoi*), people in their prime (*akmazontes*)').[42]

There is, fundamentally, a continuum between the predominant qualities of the ambient air and those of human bodies – both being understood in terms of heat, moisture and the opposites of these. And there is thus an interplay – one with potentially dramatic consequences for health – between the shifts in these qualities due to a particular season and the shifts due to an individual's age. Indeed, this parallelism between the larger time-scale of the human life and the smaller one of the yearly cycle can be extended still further in the microcosmic direction: as we shall see below, some medical authors divided the individual *day* into four parts, again following a progression in terms of successive increase and then diminution of heat (see n. 55).

In more detail, two other central Hippocratic texts, *The Nature of the Human Being* and *Aphorisms*, outline, respectively, the fundamental relationship between the seasons and the physical qualities predominant in the body and the specific diseases likely to arise in each case.

It will be worth quoting the relevant passage from the former text at some length (though with some abridgements).[43]

> Phlegm increases in the human being in winter: of the components of the body this is naturally closest to winter; for it is the coldest ... In spring the phlegm remains strong in the body, and the blood increases; for cold is reduced and the water takes its place, and blood is increased by rains and hot weather; for it is naturally closest to this time of year, since it [blood] is wet and hot. In spring and summer people fall victim to dysentery and nosebleeds, and become very hot and red. In summer the blood is still strong, and the bile is raised up in the body, extending also into autumn. In autumn blood becomes small in quantity, for the autumn is opposite to its nature; and bile dominates the body in summer and autumn. ... There is spontaneous vomiting of bile at this season, as well as vomiting induced by drugs; and it is clear also from the fevers and the complexions. Phlegm is weakest in summer: for this is the season most opposite to it, being dry and hot. Blood is least in autumn: for autumn is dry and already begins to cool the human being down. Black bile is

---

41 *Epidemics* 1.1–3, 146–52 Loeb (II.598–614 L.); The text begins: 'In Thasos, in autumn, around the equinox and near the setting of the Pleiades ...'
42 *Epidemics* 1.1, 148 Loeb (II.602 L.).
43 We may also mention the connection between diseases patterns and seasons made in *Airs, Waters, Places* 11, 52–4 Diller (II.52 L.) where the rising of the Dogstar and of Arcturus, and then the setting of the Pleiades, are stated as times when diseases especially reach their crisis.

greatest and strongest in the autumn. When winter takes hold, the bile is cooled and decreases, while the phlegm increases because of the abundance of rain and the length of the nights.

The human body always has all these, but through the changing seasons they alternate in their relative amounts, in turn, according to their nature. ... Throughout the year, first winter dominates, then spring, then summer, then autumn; so too in the human being, first phlegm dominates, then blood, then bile, first the yellow, then what is called black. The clearest evidence of this is that if you were to give the same person the same drug four times in the year, in the winter he would vomit extremely phlegmatic stuffs, in the spring extremely wet ones, in the summer extremely bilious, in the winter extremely black.[44]

In a way related to this picture, then, not only will certain diseases be more likely to arise at certain times of year, but, more broadly, provisions for diet and lifestyle in general should change cyclically in the course of the year.

Details of seasonally adjusted dietary and exercise prescriptions are given in another text, *Regimen in Health*,[45] and also in the passage already cited above from *Regimen*. Another passage, from *Aphorisms* (while in a sense elaborating in more detail the discussion just quoted from *The Nature of the Human Being*) outlines the connections between different times of year and different pathologies. Let us consider each of these in turn.

The first two chapters of *Regimen in Health* summarize the recommended diet for different times of the year, in accordance with allopathic principles, based on the perceived qualities of each season. The cold, wet nature of winter should be counteracted by plentiful roast foods and bread, and very small amounts of vegetables, and by undiluted wine, drunk in small quantities, all of which should have a drying and heating effect. In spring, drink should be increased and the foods made softer, with a reduction of the bread; all foods should be soft in summer, and the amount of water in the wine increased; a transition in the opposite direction, towards drier foods (more bread and roast foods) should take place in autumn, and so on; throughout, one must also take care to make the transitions gradual, avoiding sudden changes. Seasonally related recommendations follow regarding exercise (chs. 3 and 7) and regarding the use of emetics or enemas (ch. 5); there are also, again, remarks which make a connection between different dietary recommendations and levels of heat, dryness, etc., and different ages (chs. 2 and 6).

The passage from *Regimen* 3.68 already considered above for its statement of the fundamental division of the year gives similarly detailed dietary and exercise

---

44 *The Nature of the Human Being* 7, 182–6 Jouanna (VI.47–50 L.).
45 Known alternatively as chapters 16–24 of *The Nature of the Human Being*.

prescriptions for the four seasons; but here there is some additional, rather complex subdivision of each. Winter is divided further into a period of 44 days leading up to the winter solstice and certain periods of days after that; and spring is subdivided into even smaller units, with different recommendations for each. Here an underlying principle seems to be the importance of gradual change in the archetypally transitional period of spring.

The passage from *Aphorisms*, finally, is worth quoting *in extenso*, summarizing as it does the range of specific ailments associated with each season:

> All diseases arise at all seasons, but some tend to arise more, and to become intensified, in some seasons rather than in others. In spring, most numerous are those related to melancholy, mania and epilepsy, as well as flows of blood, sore throats, colds, hoarseness, coughing, *leprai*, *leichēnes*, *alphoi*, ulcerous *exanthēseis* [i. e., various kinds of skin complaint and pustule], growths and illnesses of the joints. In summer, some of the above, as well as continuous fevers, burning fevers, tertian fevers, vomiting, diarrhoea, eye infections, earaches, ulcers of the mouth, putrefaction of the genitals, and heat spots. In autumn, many of those of the summer, as well as quartan fevers, irregular fevers, problems of the spleen, dropsy, wasting, strangury, *leienteria* [non-absorption of food], dysentery, throat problems, asthma, ileus, epilepsy and the ailments related to mania and melancholy. In winter, pleuritis, peripneumonia, colds, lethargy, hoarseness, coughing, pains in the chest, sides and lower back, headaches, dizziness and apoplexy.[46]

Turning again to Galen, it is informative to observe both how he engages with this Hippocratic background and how seasonal factors impinge on his reported clinical experience and practice.

On a theoretical level, first: while Galen purports to be in full agreement with the views of 'Hippocrates', which he takes to be represented by both *The Nature of the Human Being* and the *Aphorisms*, he in fact departs from the position clearly implied by these, namely that each season of the year is in its own way equally pathological. In his major treatise on related themes, *Mixtures*, Galen argues at length against doctors who make precisely this mistake; in this context, indeed, he explicitly accuses of them of seeking to find a correspondence between each season and an unbalanced state – that is, of striving for precisely the kind of artificially neat correspondence which we have noted from time to time throughout this chapter.[47] Spring, he insists, is *not* 'hot' or 'wet' in the same sense that those terms are used in relation to the other seasons to which they are applied – that is, to indicate an excess. There is, in fact, no season which is both hot and wet in

---

46 *Aphorisms* 3.19–23, 128–20 Loeb (IV.494–6 L.).
47 See especially the argument of *Mixtures* 1.4, where he attacks 'the desire to find the fourth pairing of mixtures in the seasons at all costs', 10 Helmreich (I.524 K.).

that sense – in the sense of naturally giving rise to diseases arising from heat and moisture. Spring, rather, is warm and moist, but healthily so: it is the season of good balance, possessed of precisely the right degree of both heat and moisture.

Whatever the precise nature of his relationship with the Hippocratic tradition, however, seasonal differences play a major role in Galen's assessment of human health and its management. In the realm of the maintenance of health, many examples could be given of the tailoring of diet and exercise to the seasons, along similar lines to that observed in *Regimen* and *Regimen in Health*, above: predominances of particular physical qualities, and of the related fluids, at different seasons are frequently presented as predisposing causes or exacerbating factors, especially where the person in question already suffers from a predominance of the fluid in question (e.g. phlegm, in winter); these should lead to a prescription of diet and exercise designed to bring about the opposite qualities.

At the level of actual disease, too, there are close connections between different seasons and different predominant pathologies, again with related precautions and interventions to be undertaken. Let us give just a few examples.

Fevers – that central category in ancient medicine, to which we shall return in more detail in chapter 4 – are differentially related to the different fluids that predominate in the body, and thus – as we would expect on the basis of the kind of analysis we have seen above – also to the different seasons and different times of life. Each of the main types of intermittent fever is related to the predominance of one type of fluid. (The situation regarding the fourth main type, the continuous fever, is rather more complicated.) Here too, incidentally, Galen explicitly departs from the model of rival doctors – which again has Hippocratic authority – according to which fevers in general are produced by excess yellow bile. Galen's typology by contrast is summarized in Table 5.[48]

---

48 *The Nature of the Human Being* states that most fevers, which are four in type, arise from bile, differing in the *amount* of bile involved, although it does go on to admit that the quartan involves also an *admixture* of black bile: 15, 202–4 Jouanna (VI.66–8 L.). The table summarizes Galen's argument in *The Distinct Types of Fever* 2.1 (VII.333–6 K.), where he also explicitly attacks those who attribute fevers in general to yellow bile.

TABLE 5: Galen's typology of fevers

Fever type	Dominant fluid	Life stage	Season	Environment or external influence
quotidian	phlegm	children and old people	winter	cold and wet
tertian	yellow bile	prime	summer	hot and dry
quartan	black bile	post-prime	autumn	cold and dry

It this context of our consideration of the ways in which the two cycles, that of the seasons and that of ages, are explicitly connected with each other by Galen (and also of the relationship of this Galenic discourse to the Hippocratic one) it is informative to note a passage in *The Doctrines of Hippocrates and Plato* – where, indeed, Galen quotes at length several of the Hippocratic passages which we have considered in this chapter. After citing that from *The Nature of Man*, he adds: 'by making these statements about the difference in the seasons, Hippocrates taught us *by implication* about the differences in times of life and regions' (8.6, 516 De Lacy, V.692 K.). Galen is keen to establish that the remarks in this text about seasonal difference belong within the broader picture which he himself espouses, whereby predominant fluid, time of year and age are conceptually linked.[49]

Relatedly, different clinical outcomes will be anticipated at different seasons: Galen mentions the case of Eudemus, 'who was suffering from three quartan fevers in the middle of winter, and had been despaired of by his doctors'.[50] Galen successfully supervises and predicts his recovery, but the expectation, on the basis of the time of year, was clearly a negative one.

A further example throws into vivid relief the perceived effect of the seasonal cycle on health and disease. Galen recounts the case of a sufferer from melancholy who would come to him regularly every year, at the moment when he first became aware of the onset of symptoms, in order to have Galen perform the appropriate purgative treatment to remove black bile. People who regularly 'evacuate their own residues every spring or autumn' through a variety of medicines, both laxative and emetic, are also mentioned.[51] The examples highlight

---

[49] Further explicit Galenic links could be mentioned too: differences in the pulse can be broadly categorized according to both age and season (*The Pulse for Beginners* 9).
[50] *Prognosis* 3, 82 Nutton (XIV.613 K.).
[51] See *Commentary on Hippocrates' Aphorisms* 1.67 (XVIIIA.79 K.); *Health* 4.4, 107 Koch (VI.244 K.).

the prominence of the seasonal cycle in the perception of illness, not just on the part of the doctor but also on that of the patient.

Non-periodic disease recurrence: some endless cycles

Finally, two further types of disease pattern should be mentioned which, though they are less clearly connected with a regular temporal cycle, recur on a chronic or intermittent basis. They are two which also had a widespread and dramatic effect on people's lives, even though it is one which we glimpse only faintly, through the few Galenic texts which briefly mention them.

One is the Antonine Plague, which affected the population of Rome catastrophically, and intermittently, for a considerable period of years, from its first outbreak in 165 CE, when it was brought to the city by troops returning from the near east. In this case, the relationship of the disease to time seems to be marked rather by its lack of certainty or precision. Galen's few references to the plague – after his first mention of its initial outbreak, at which he returned in haste to his homeland of Pergamum – are to something which is long, and apparently ongoing; they emphasize its intractability, the impossibility of defining it terms of a clear timespan or duration. Nor, though there are intermittent outbreaks, is there any regularity – nothing that can be tied to cycle of seasons. He speaks of 'the plague which arose, and continues', of 'the long-running plague', of 'the very long plague which arose in our time', of 'one fierce outbreak of the long-running plague'. It is something unpredictable and variable, but apparently – at the time of most of his references to it – permanently with us. Nor does he omit to comment at that first reference to it that it is untreatable: 'no one had been able to find a powerful enough drug to combat this scourge, which spread everywhere before being extinguished'.[52]

Doubtless the plague had some relationship to the cycle of the seasons (the first, most virulent outbreak took place in the winter) but it appears in Galen's few mentions rather as a disease without temporal markers – almost, a timeless disease, a perpetual affliction.

---

52 *My Own Books* 1, 139 Boudon-Millot (XIX.15 K.); *Prognosis by the Pulse* 3.4 (IX.357 K.); *Commentary on Hippocrates' Epidemics, book 3* 3.76, 163 Wenkebach and Pfaff (XVIIA.741 K.); *Avoiding Distress* 1, 2,6–7 BJP. (The final remark, on its untreatability, appears in the first text cited, where however it is absent from the Greek text and supplied on the basis of the Arabic translation; see Boudon-Millot ad loc.) On Galen's discussion of the plague, as well as further analysis of its history and possible microbiological identity, see Flemming (2019).

The second disease pattern is visible even more faintly in the Galenic text, although it again was surely something that involved widespread suffering. In a discussion of the effects of different foodstuffs on health, Galen remarks:

> In many regions under Roman rule, the inhabitants of the cities, whose procedure is always, at the end of summer, to lay up a sufficient store of grain for the whole of the following year, remove from the farms all the wheat, barley, beans and lentils, and leave the rural population the remaining crops, which are known as cereals and pulses (as well as taking to the city a considerable quantity even of these). What is left to the locals is quickly exhausted, so that they are compelled throughout the whole spring to consume shoots of trees and shrubs, as well as bulbs and roots of plants which have poor humoral fluid; they fill themselves also with wild vegetables, as they are known, of which they may be fortunate enough to have a plentiful supply, and also cook and eat certain fresh green plants, which they have never before even tasted, whole. By the end of spring some of them, and by the beginning of summer nearly all, would be observed to be affected by copious ulcerations on the skin ...[53]

After describing a range of presentations and pathological outcomes of these, he concludes:

> In some, they become carbuncular and tumorous and, in conjunction with fever, lead to the death of the sufferers, over a long period, with very few being saved, and those with great difficulty.[54]

There are, moreover, fevers and digestive problems which arise, with fatal consequences, even in the absence of the skin complaints. The passage continues with further details of anomalous foodstuffs and their dangerous consequences.

Galen's argumentative purpose in this text is simply to demonstrate 'what great power bad humoral fluid (*kakochumia*) has to bring about diseases', as he says right at the beginning of the whole passage (and indeed the treatise), just before the first extract quoted above. That is, he is keen to assert the validity and importance of his Hippocratically based humoral model of explanation of nutrition, health and disease, and the dangers that arise when doctors reject this model.

In passing, however, and as it were by accident, he has opened a window on a world of endemic malnutrition, a world in which certain diseases, some fatal,

---

53 *Good and Bad Humoral Fluid* 1, 389 Helmreich (VI.749–50 K.). The precise identity of the grains or pulses taken or left, as also that of the variety of wild plants consumed, cannot be ascertained; the picture is however clearly one in which the higher-quality crops are taken and the inferior ones left, and these in insufficient quantity.
54 Ibid. 390 Helmreich (VI.350–1 K.).

tend to recur on a seasonal basis, as a function of an agricultural economy which imposes and perpetuates a dramatic inequality between a city-dwelling elite and the rural population.

Conclusion regarding medical discussions of cycles

A recurrent theme that has arisen in our consideration of medical and other theoretical accounts, both of the times of life and of the seasons of the year, is the interplay between the ambition to produce theoretical neatness or symmetry, on the one hand, and the conclusions of more open-ended or empirically based discussions, on the other.

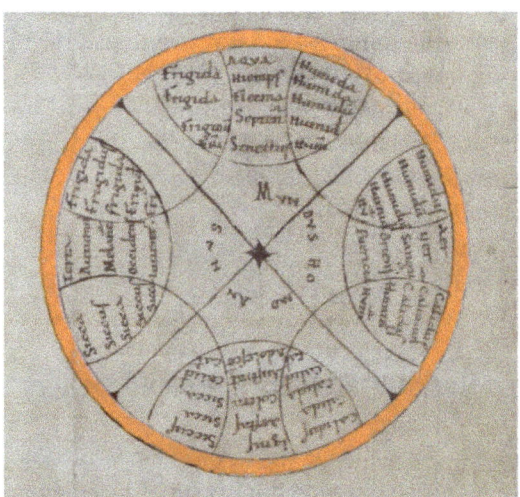

Figure 9: 'Mundus homo annus': the mediaeval circle of correspondences of elements, seasons, fluids and ages. Such circular images, representing a range of correspondences in microcosm and macrocosm, became common in mediaeval medical and scientific texts (though the correspondences in some respects represent a departure from the Galenic view). This one is from a manuscript of Bede's *De temporum ratione*, MS Sankt Gallen, Stiftsbibliothek, 248, f. 148. Image source: https://link.springer.com/article/10.1007/s40656-021-00425-3

The diagram in figure 9 represents a series of correspondences, and a theoretical consensus, which enjoyed considerable prominence in post-Galenic medicine, for a number of centuries. Here each of the four elements is connected with one of the four seasons, one of the four bodily fluids (humours), one of the four ages and, in some cases, one of the four points of the compass. For clarification, the correspondences in question are listed in Table 6.

TABLE 6: The mediaeval circle of correspondences: 'world – man – year'

Water (cold/wet)	Air (wet/hot)	Fire (hot/dry)	Earth (dry/cold)
Winter	Spring	Summer	Autumn
Phlegm	Blood	Bile	Black bile (melancholy)
North	East	South	West
Old Age	Childhood	Youth (*adulescentia*)	Young adulthood (*iuventus*)

Such a table or circle of correspondences also represents a rationalizing project, an attempt at neatness or simplification, which will be tendentially impervious to empirical inputs or adjustments. In this context, it is noteworthy that Galen disagrees with the information represented here in at least two important respects, both of which have been observed in the course of this chapter. First, he insists that old age is dry, not wet. Secondly, he denies that spring corresponds to the departures from good balance involved in the other seasons, by being 'hot and wet'. Thus, Galen insists, on the basis of his clinical observations, on two crucial departures from this abstract rationalization – and does so in spite of what seems to have been a substantial consensus in its favour, a consensus also with at least some claim to Hippocratic authority.[55]

A final consideration: temporal and atemporal human beings

The model whereby all human beings are positioned within one of four (or more) life stages, of roughly equal length, itself raises a fundamental question of human self-perception. To what extent do human beings experience themselves as constantly temporally determined in this way – or to what extent are they so regarded by their society? According to the schemes considered above, the neutral term *anēr*, and the temporally related one *akmazōn*, correspond simply to

---

[55] Further correspondences are possible, again representing a departure from or variation upon the familiar Hippocratic or 'Galenic' theme. Fragments of the (probably) first/second-century-CE medical authors Athenaeus of Attalia and Antyllus advance the view that the day may be divided into four parts, in a sense representing a microcosm of the four seasons: dawn is wet and hot like spring, the middle of the day like summer, the afternoon or evening like autumn, and the night like winter; and these differences again have implications for the appropriateness of medical interventions. (The former is quoted in Aëtius of Amida, *Medical Books* 3.162,29–35; the latter in Stobaeus, *Anthology* 4.37.15.)

stages in a constantly changing cycle. Yet, in another sense, this stage corresponds rather to the true or full instantiation of the human self. In that sense, this adult or mature version of the human being may be considered rather as its correct or normal physical version, rather than as simply one stage amongst others. It may be the stage at which one ideally imagines oneself, both in anticipation as a child or youth, and after the stage has in fact biologically passed.

It may be fruitful in this context to consider portraiture, and in particular the age – or lack of it – at which an individual in elite society chooses to have him- or herself depicted or memorialized. Might it be said that the portrait images made of Roman noblemen and emperors, at whatever actual age they are made, correspond to 'atemporal' or ideal selves? That it is an ideal age, or a transcendence of age, that is being represented, rather than a biologically specific time of life?[56]

A huge literature surrounds the question of how to 'read' Roman portrait statues, as well as their complex stylistic historical developments. Without venturing too deeply into these areas, we may at least observe that two apparently conflicting dynamics are in play in the Roman Republic and early empire, both of which, however, are relevant to our discussion. On the one hand, we have the supposedly 'veristic' portrait sculptures of the Republican period, which seem to represent people burdened with all the attributes of middle or old age, on the other the type especially associated with Augustus, whereby the emperor continues, throughout his life (and beyond it) to be represented as a man in extreme youth. The latter more obviously suggests the choice of an ideal age, or a state of agelessness, as corresponding to the true self that the patron wishes to have represented in his images; it can also be seen as a departure from the aged or timebound images of the Republican great and good that preceded it. One might, however, alternatively argue that *both* the 'veristic' Republican type *and* the Augustan permanent youth represent the choice of an ideal age, which stands outside the actual passage of time – especially when once one accepts modern scholarly cautions as to the nature of the chronological 'realism', as opposed to designed symbolism, involved in the former.[57] That is to say, the apparently realistic self-images of the middle-aged or aged Republican states-

---

56 The point is suggested by Laurence (2000).
57 In a classic discussion, Nodelman (1993) argued against the reading of Republican portraits as 'realistic', pointing to the symbolic value, and clearly chosen nature, of their many recurrent physiognomic features: deep lines and sunken eyes signify moral seriousness, self-restraint and statesmanlike virtue, not simple biological age. For wide-ranging accounts of the stylistic developments and portrait types see further Fejfer (2008); La Rocca and Parisi Presicce (2011); and for a survey of recent literature Borg (2012).

men also involve the choice of an ideal age, or of ideal, time-transcending attributes, with which they choose to be depicted or immortalized.

One may, equally, contrast the biologically or temporally determined account of the human life with views of the self that arise in the philosophical tradition, as well as with those implied by certain tendencies in ancient biography. The latter – and the tension that arises between atemporal and chronologically conditioned selves in that context – will be explored further in the next chapter. With regard to the former, discussion of ancient views of the self, and of their relationship to a physically fluctuating body, is beyond my scope here. It may however be observed, at least, that – to give just one example – a Platonic view of the self in terms of an essentially atemporal soul which *uses* or *inhabits* the body, and which moreover strives to minimize the extent to which it is conditioned by that body, will tend to give a fundamentally different perspective on the nature of the constantly shifting cycle than those implied by the medical perspectives considered above.

Chapter Three:
Lives in time: history, biography, bibliography

In this chapter I explore two related themes, reflecting on aspects of Graeco-Roman self-perception and self-presentation. First, I ask what conception Roman imperial – and to an extent also earlier – authors have of distinct periods of previous history, and of the period to which they themselves belong. Secondly, how do they chronicle or periodize their own lives or life's work: to what extent is such chronicling tied to particular moments or dates, and to what extent aiming at an atemporal perspective, transcending their own time or indeed time-based narrative altogether?

The second topic could be considered from a number of further perspectives, which I only touch on here. Some of these perspectives are however worth mentioning briefly before proceeding, as suggesting further relevant background to our enquiry. I refer to the perspectives offered by horoscopal astrology; by the recording of human lifespans, as evidenced by funerary inscriptions; and by philosophical reflections on the passing of time and the appropriate attitude to it.

In astrology, it was considered important to know the precise hour of the birth in order to cast a horoscope successfully; a preoccupation with astrology will thus have contributed to the desire or need to record birth times with precision.[1]

As regards funerary inscriptions, it is striking that a number of gravestones record the lifespan of the deceased in terms not just of years, months and days, but also of hours, and sometimes even fractions of hours. We note the occurrence of the term *scrupulus*, usually used for a very small weight, but here referring to a period of a 24th of an hour. The practice seems especially prevalent in cases of loss of a child, the authors of these intensely poignant memorials seemingly exercised to cling on to every last moment of the life that has gone, and such a full numerical account somehow contributing to the memorialization of the life of the departed loved one. (See figure 10.) So, to look at just a few striking cases:[2]

---

[1] See Barton (1994a), (1994b) and (1995), the latter two works in particular laying out the complexities and variety of relevant information potentially relevant to the casting of horoscopes, including that of the emperor Augustus; specifically on the astrological demand for precision in relation to birth time, see Heilen (2020).
[2] The texts are taken from the collection of such precise-lifespan memorials assembled and discussed by Luciani (2009). (See further Ehrlich 2012.) The first three are from Rome, the fourth from Pisa and the fifth from Numidia, and all date from somewhere between the second and

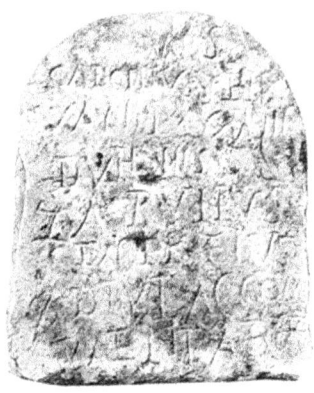

Figure 10: A Roman funerary inscription recording a lifespan of 75 years, 3 months, 5 days, 3-and-a-half hours (Luciani 2009, no. 11). Image source: Corbier and Gascou (1995), 280, https://www.persee.fr/doc/antaf_0066-4871_1995_num_31_1_1239

Abuccius Silvanus lived 3 years, 6 months, 29 days and 6-and-a-half hours.
To Cornelia Thymele, their beloved daughter, her most unhappy parents.
Calpurnius Diceus and Secura. She lived 7 years, 2 months, 19 days and an hour and a half.
Eleutera lived 3 years, 28 days, 2-and-a-half hours.
To the deserving Silvana, who sleeps here, in peace. She lived 21 years, 3 months, 4 hours, 6 *scrupuli*.

Such monuments are not however confined to the very young; there is at least one opposite case, where precision contributes to the commemoration of a very long life:

Caecilius Felix lived 75 years, 3 months, 5 days, 3-and-a-half hours.

It is noteworthy, meanwhile, that such personal monuments in general do not, unlike their modern counterparts, contain *dating*, that is, any indication linking those years, months or hours to externally fixed points – a procedure which would be of relevance rather to the first of our two questions, that of the self-contextualization of ancient lives. Such dating – which typically functions by mentioning officials serving at a particular time, in the Roman world usually the consuls – tends to feature rather only in inscriptions of a public nature, those which proclaim a law, commemorate a victor, or dedicate a monument in the name the benefactor. The private time of these monuments of indi-

---

the fourth century CE. They appear there as nos. 3, 6, 20, 22 and 11. The practice seems common to pagan and Christian memorials of the period: the first two and the last cited here are pagan, the remaining two Christian. (For a much more comprehensive account of the recording of lifespans on Roman inscriptions, specifically Christian context, see Nordberg 1963.)

vidual lives seems thus to exist in a separate realm from that of public events, appointments and calendars.³

The evidence for both these preoccupations, that of horoscope-casting and that of the recording of the precise number of hours of a life, casts further light on the question considered in chapter 1, of the role of time-telling technologies in everyday lives. Indeed, it seems to suggest a significantly widespread role for these technologies, at least in certain critical contexts – the moments of birth and death. (It may very well indeed be that the two are intimately connected, that is, that the popular motivation for a close attention to the hour of birth, in particular, was, precisely, an astrological one.)

Meanwhile philosophers, especially Stoic ones, offer further perspectives on – and to some extent reversals of – popular attitudes to the valuing of the days and hours of a life, and to the human lifespan as a whole. And the 'modern' time-telling technology of the water-clock has a strong relevance here too. In Petronius' *Satyricon* the rich host Trimalchio is introduced as an 'exquisite fellow, with a clock in his dining room, and a trumpeter, so that he may always know how much life he has lost'; here the picture is a satirical one, although it presumably at some level reflects a genuine anxiety.⁴ The philosopher Seneca, on the other hand, while also bearing witness to this association of the draining of water from a *clepsydra* with the running-out of life, aims to transform the attendant preoccupation or anxiety: it is not the last bit of water that should concern us, the bit that has just run out; not the last moments, but the whole lifespan. Life has in fact been in a constant process of dripping away – death has been coming all along, we are dying all the time – so there is nothing special to frighten us about the last drops.⁵

Such a perception is, for Seneca, of a piece with the correct attitude to time itself, which involves a philosophically differential approach to past (to be grasped in the memory), present (to be appropriately utilized) and future (to be anticipated). The full achievement of this attitude to time indeed constitutes a liberation from normal human laws: such simultaneous mental comprehending of 'all

---

3 There are exceptions: a consulate is mentioned for example in another of the inscriptions discussed by Luciani (2009: no. 18); but such mentions seem rare.
4 Petronius, *Satyricon* 26.
5 'cotidie morimur ... tunc quoque, cum crescimus, vita decrescit ... quemadmodum clepsydram non extremum stillicidium exhaurit, sed quidquid ante defluxit, sic ultima hora, qua esse desinimus, non sola mortem facit, sed sola consummat', Seneca, *Moral Letters* 24.19–20. Water and river metaphors are widely used by Seneca to help induce the correct attitude to the flow of life, as explored by Armisen-Marchetti (1989); see further Miller (forthcoming), ch. 4.

times' is a vital attribute of the sage – one, that, in some crucial psychological sense, makes his life a long one.[6]

Other Stoic exhortatory arguments against the fear of death draw in different ways on these same notions of the fleeting nature of a life's moments, and of the relationship of these moments to the whole human lifespan. So, Epictetus encourages one not to think of oneself as eternity (*aiōn*) but rather 'as a part of the whole, as an hour is of a day; I must come about like an hour, and pass by like an hour'. Going further, Marcus Aurelius characterizes the 'time of human life' as merely a moment (*stigmē*), and describes human life as 'momentary' (*akariaios*), or a 'momentary section of eternity'.[7]

Such reflections are obviously designed to bring about a re-evaluation of our lives, based precisely on their temporal insignificance: our human lifespans are as nothing when considered in relation to eternity. Marcus, building on the Epictetan dictum that 'you can only lose what you have', elaborates a further argument, which can be summarized as follows. All that you *have* is the present (*to paron*), which is further characterized as 'momentary' (*akariaion*); in dying, therefore, you are losing neither past nor future; everyone who dies, then, loses exactly the same thing, namely that single, momentary present; so, considerations of the length, or nature, of the life previously lived, as well as considerations of a hypothetical future lost, are irrelevant.[8]

---

6 'transit tempus aliquod? – hoc recordatione comprendit. instat? – hoc utitur. venturum est? – hoc praecipit. longam illi vitam facit omnium temporum in unum conlatio', Seneca, *The Brevity of Life* 15.5. For analysis of this Senecan process of mental mastery or 'appropriation' of time, past, present and future, see Armisen-Marchetti (1995).
7 Arrian, *Discourses of Epictetus* 2.5.13; Marcus Aurelius, *Meditations* 2.17; 2.6; 11.8; 5.24; cf. 3.36, where 'all present time is a moment of eternity'. For philosophical views of the nature of eternity itself see further below, chapter 5.
8 *Meditations* 2.14; cf. 3.10. Marcus' temporally-based argument, like Epictetus', is fundamentally instrumental or therapeutic in its nature, and does not engage explicitly with theoretical analyses of time, of the sort which had been given in earlier Stoicism (and into which I also do not enter here); it has attracted some criticism on the grounds of its alleged theoretical inadequacy. See Mouroutsou (2020) for a survey of previous literature and a theoretical defence of Marcus' position, based on the understanding of the present as 'plastic' (i.e. flexible in its precise extension) and of the verb 'have' in the above argument as crucially connected to what is 'up to us' in the Stoic sense: that is, what it means that we 'have' the present is precisely that our action within that present is under our control. Whatever its strengths or weaknesses when subjected to such analysis, however, it is the mental attitude aimed at, and the relationship of that to the attitudes abroad in Marcus' society, that concern us here. (There is, clearly, a potential connection between the argument discussed and the paradox of the 'ceasing instant', which we shall consider (albeit fleetingly) in chapter 5, although such a connection is not developed by Marcus.)

The mental reduction of our experienced lives to the present moment is not just of value in relation to the contemplation of death. Elsewhere, Marcus tells himself not to be led astray by 'a mental impression (*phantasia*) of your whole life', including the nature and magnitude of worries past and future, and to remind himself that it is, in fact, only the present that has the capacity to cause distress (since grief for the past and worry about the future are in fact both *present* events); moreover, the precise scope of this present can be diminished (*katasmikrunetai*) by mental exercise. Still more positively, Marcus cajoles his soul to be satisfied with its true nature, in need of nothing external – and in particular to be satisfied with the *present* state and not feel the need for more *time*.[9]

The perception that all you lose at death is a single 'moment' – that the present moment is, in some psychologically important sense, all that a human life is – may seem opposed in its tendency to Seneca's perception, just considered, that past, present and future in a life should all be appropriately valued, or to his claim that a life is conceptually made 'long' by such mental mastery. But both kinds of perception can perhaps be united within a broader view, or better, a broader recommended psychological approach. This approach is concerned above all to value the present moment, and in particular, the opportunity it brings for correct action and attitude, while not, however, being attached to the notion of the continuance of that moment into the future. At the same time, however – in that same moment, indeed – one may derive benefit from thoughts of both past and future, provided that such thoughts do not include a hankering after, or revived distress at, what has passed, on the one hand, or a preoccupation with future states which may or may not eventuate, on the other.

Whether we find the attitudes encouraged by these Stoic authors valuable, helpful, or indeed possible, the texts cited in their own way also bespeak – through their very attempts to counter it – a preoccupation with the constant passing of time and constantly diminishing available human lifespan, and to an extent also a preoccupation with its measurement.

My investigation in this chapter, however, will have a more specifically literary–intellectual focus, as opposed to one based in either broader perceptions or life practices, on the one hand, or philosophical speculations or recommendations, on the other. I shall consider these questions – that of the attitude to the past and that of the chronicling of lives – in the particular context of Roman imperial writing. And I shall take as my case study for the investigation the works of, and attitudes exemplified by, Galen – the author who gives fuller

---

[9] *Meditations* 8.36; 10.1; the focus on the now and rejection of considerations of past and future recurs also at 12.3.

evidence than any other imperial-period author of both literary biography and bibliographical practice, while also being a *par excellence* representative of the classicizing literary and intellectual culture of his times, the so-called 'Second Sophistic'.

The old and the new

We live in times far removed from the golden age of which our elders dream, of which the fables tell. The perception is a recurrent one, in a variety of cultures and chronological periods. In the Graeco-Roman world, its most famous version is, precisely, that of the mythical Golden Race, of which we are the distant and decadent successors.[10] But it finds its counterpart in intellectual history too.

Both the scientific and the literary culture of the first centuries of our era were in a sense extremely backward-looking – based in an education in the language and literature of an age long past, looking to the classical greats of that past for inspiration and support, tending to prefer the authority of the old to the appeal of the new. The origins of this culture, or classicizing tendency, may themselves be traced to a period several centuries earlier, to the Hellenizing culture that took root from the third century BCE, and of which the Museum and Library of Alexandria were the most outstanding representative. It was at this period – and at this location especially – that a core set of 'classical' texts was established, and practices of scholarship and criticism developed, that remained central to the education and literary culture even of Galen's time. There, then, if not before, we begin to find a distinction in the intellectual and literary context, between a previous, 'classical' age and the one we presently inhabit.

Within that Hellenistic era itself, the classicizing tendency held sway mainly in the area of literary texts. True, the same bibliophile techniques of scholarship

---

[10] See Hesiod, *Works and Days* 109–201. The first race of humans was the golden one (109); ours, that of iron (176), is at four removes from it (after the silver, the bronze, and that of the heroes); and even this will become so decadent that it will be destroyed by a worse one (180–201). In the better-known version of Ovid (*Metamorphoses* 1.89–150) the present race, that of iron, is at three removes from the first (after silver and bronze). For further ancient versions, including parallel myths in other cultures, and for analysis of the Hesiodic account, see Most (1997). Most argues for a closer potential connection between the present race and that of the heroes, and a less inevitable and absolute decline, than one takes from a surface reading of the text; whether or not one finds that interpretation convincing, it seems clear that the myth was standardly understood in the ancient world in terms of irredeemable present-day decadence.

and criticism came to be applied also to 'ancient' scientific or medical texts, in particular those of the so-called Hippocratic corpus: indeed, it was at this period that such a corpus first came to be assembled, with a range of texts for various reasons attributed to the famous historical figure of Hippocrates.[11] But, for most of the Hellenistic period, at least, the interest in these was, precisely, a historical one: the texts were the subject of antiquarian or scholarly research, but were not at this stage taken as authoritative in any scientific sense. The notion, still familiar to us today, of Hippocrates as 'father of medicine' – and even, indeed, the notion that his work was in any important scientific sense different in kind from that of a range of other medical authors, of whom there were also extant texts – were to come much later. Moreover, this same period of the third and second centuries BCE was one of considerable medical *innovation* at Alexandria, by anatomical researchers such as Herophilus and Erasistratus, in particular (on whom, more later).

Things had changed by Galen's time. At some point – albeit not in a way that commanded universal agreement – Hippocrates had ceased to be *merely* a focus of historical and scholarly interest and become *also* a source of medical authority. In Galen's medical education, and most prominently of all within his own subsequent practice, scholarship and science are fused: empirically based arguments for the truth of a particular medical view fade into scholarly arguments for the proposition that Hippocrates espoused that view too, and vice versa.[12] Such arguments, as one would expect in relation to texts of a period more than 500 years before one's own – a 500 years which have seen major advances, especially in anatomy – rely on a highly sophisticated repertory of scholarly and interpretive techniques and approaches. Techniques and approaches, indeed, which closely parallel those which, from late antique to contemporary times, have enabled members of particular religious communities to discern their own theological and philosophical views in biblical texts that belong to an age, and a social and intellectual context, far distant from their own

Such classicizing developments in medicine are, in very broad terms, paralleled by those in philosophy. Here too, while there were major innovations in the Hellenistic period, the main philosophical schools were established by the first century CE. Of course, there continue to be significant further innovations and original discussions, but from this point on these arise largely in a process of dia-

---

11 See von Staden (1992), (2006); more broadly on the history of the 'invention of Hippocrates', Smith (1979).
12 On this cultural background and Galen's place in it see especially Lloyd (1993), von Staden (2004), (2009).

logue with and commentary on an existing body of texts, itself regarded as in some sense classical and authoritative.

More broadly, and if one considers Roman alongside Greek literary culture, Latin authors famously conceived their great works as closely modelled on the great Greek classics. Here too, originality lies in adaptation and transformation; innovation is often concealed behind the claim to be following in ancient footsteps. We shall pursue this theme – and the related one of the potentially atemporal self-image of the author – with a particular focus on Galen, who is one of the most prolific as well as most revealing representatives of the Greek literary culture of the Roman period, though we shall end the chapter with a comparison of Galen's attitude and self-positioning with those of another major intellectual and biographer of the imperial period, Porphyry. The themes investigated here could, of course, be considered in relation to a range of other imperial-period authors; I offer the analysis here as one which is both potentially representative of imperial literary and intellectual culture, on the one hand, and suggestive of further lines of research, on the other.[13]

Galen on the old and the new (1): the ideology of the ancient

A central theme in Galen's work, arising constantly in his references to predecessors, is the distinction between 'ancients', *palaioi* and 'younger' or 'more recent', *neōteroi*, authors, doctors especially. Neither term is completely univocal or straightforward in its reference; and there is, I shall argue, more than one conception of past time, and of self-positioning in relation to it, in play here.

As has been highlighted by much recent scholarship, Galen's approach to the previous tradition – connected with that culture of the Second Sophistic – is an archaizing or classicizing one, in which he both elevates the contribution of the great 'ancients', Hippocrates and Plato in particular, and presents himself as their avatar or equal, by contrast despising or neglecting the decadent *neōteroi*.[14] This perception is undoubtedly true, as is the tendentially transtemporal view of Galen that emerges from it. At the same time – and in a way that has not been similarly acknowledged by scholarship – Galen presents us, alongside this idealistically and ideologically loaded view of past and present time, with a

---

13 On this literary and intellectual culture more broadly see Swain (1996); Goldhill (2001); Whitmarsh (2001); Richter and Johnson (2017).
14 See von Staden (1997); Vegetti (2001); more broadly on Galen's position in this cultural and intellectual landscape Gill, Whitmarsh and Wilkins (2009); Singer (2013): 4–17; (2014); (2019a); Mattern (2017).

much more historiographically neutral, indeed chronologically quite sophisticated, attempt at the periodization of past time. We shall proceed to examine both aspects of this Galenic historiography in what follows; the terms 'ancient' and 'more recent' are used in a fluid and shifting way – but nevertheless with distinctly identifiable senses according to different contexts – throughout Galen's work.

To begin, then, with Galen's idealized view of the past and the 'ancients'. We shall talk further about the precise reference, or references, of the term *palaios* below; but underlying the terminology is, almost always, a sense of the 'golden age' which is, in a way, the counterpart in intellectual history of the Hesiodic golden age mentioned above. Indeed Galen even, as we shall see shortly, makes explicit reference to Hesiod's golden age in his characterization of the classical period of Greek medicine. Broadly speaking, however, we may say that by *palaioi* Galen means, on the medical side, above all Hippocrates, and on the philosophical side, above all Plato; but that further respected ancients may be added on both sides: on the former, such post-Hippocratic authorities as Diocles or Praxagoras: on the latter, Aristotle and Theophrastus, and sometimes even Stoics. In fact, Galen constructs a shifting 'line of authority' (in Vegetti's phrase), assembling the maximum number of potentially respectable authority figures that can be called upon in support of any given position – and attacking others who ignore such an impressive display – even if some of these authority figures are individuals (like Chrysippus, Praxagoras, or even Aristotle) with whom he has profound disagreements in other areas.[15]

One of Galen's most impressive works – central to his output and, arguably, that with which he made his reputation – is *The Doctrines of Hippocrates and Plato*. Both the intellectual project and its execution are quite remarkable. Here, Galen sets forth the essentials of his own physiological views on the functioning of the most important organs in the human body (the brain, the heart and the liver), on the nervous and vascular systems and on element theory.

---

15 See Vegetti (1999a), (1999b). So, for example, Plato and Aristotle are lined up against the Stoics on the issue of the fundamental division between rational and non-rational faculties or parts of the soul; Plato and Hippocrates are lined up against Aristotle, the Stoics and a range of medical authors, including Praxagoras, on the fact that the brain, not the heart, is the command-centre of the soul; Praxagoras and a large number of others are mentioned with approval (against, for example, Atomists, Methodists or Asclepiadeans) in the area of element theory and health prescriptions; even Chrysippus and the Stoics form part of the respected authority tradition in certain contexts, for example in their advocacy of a form of physicalism (in *The Soul's Dependence on the Body*); and, as we shall see, in one case even Asclepiades forms part of a near-universal consensus against Erasistratus. See further note 25 below.

And he does so on the basis of detailed reference to the most up-to-date anatomical research, and his own dramatic public anatomical (in some cases vivisectional) demonstrations used to elucidate these. At the same time, however, the central aim of the work involves the establishment of at least three propositions which are, from a modern historical perspective, frankly absurd:[16]

(1) Hippocrates and Plato were in agreement on their fundamental doctrines regarding the human body (and, in a sense, the soul)
(2) Plato was indebted to Hippocrates for these views
(3) Galen's views on anatomy and physiology were in their essentials anticipated by the ancients, by Hippocrates in particular.

And these perceptions are not just eccentricities or oddities of this work, a function of its particular purposes and stated aims – although, undoubtedly, the work is a rhetorical tour-de-force, breath-taking in the ingenuity of the arguments, and the scholarly expertise, which are marshalled in their pursuit. Rather, this self-perception and this historiographical perspective – Galen as the avatar of Hippocrates and Plato in his disinterested devotion to and assiduous pursuit of the truth, Hippocrates and Plato as anticipating Galen in the essentials of his anatomical, medical and philosophical views – run through Galen's whole career and literary output. Plato's philosophy of mind and ethics (sometimes called his moral psychology) underlie Galen's thought in those areas especially, although – as already remarked – he also claims the philosopher's agreement with the fundamentals of his own physiology of the brain, heart and liver, as well as of his element theory, and takes himself to be following Plato also in logical or scientific method. He claims Hippocrates' agreement, meanwhile, not just on the essentials of physiology but also in all matters to do with day-to-day healthcare, disease definition and clinical practice. And he does this *passim* throughout his scientific or philosophical writings on these different subjects, but also in the context of his voluminous commentaries on the Hippocratic writings, which constitute something like a third of his enormous output.[17] (We have already seen just a few examples of the tensions involved in this retrojection of his own views onto Hippocrates, in the previous chapter.)

---

[16] For analysis of the tensions that arise in this project see (alongside the work already cited of Smith, Lloyd, Vegetti and von Staden) Singer (1996), (2021).
[17] Galen also wrote commentaries on Plato and Aristotle, though none of the latter has survived, and only one of the former, in fragmentary form.

The reality is that Galen is indebted for his anatomical education and views to a much more recent tradition – and indeed, that is something which, as we shall see, he elsewhere openly admits (while never resiling from the claim that such anatomical knowledge was in some way anticipated by Hippocrates centuries earlier).[18] Yet that reality is completely obscured, put to one side, in the context of the construction of his intellectual heritage presented by *The Doctrines of Hippocrates and Plato*, and indeed in most of his major works.

This ideologically loaded approach to the history of medicine has some remarkable consequences, as already noted. Particularly striking is the construction of the intellectual and ethical milieu of the golden era of Greek medicine. This was the age of Hippocrates. One Galenic passage presents this construction of that past intellectual tradition – and disparagement of the present – with especial vividness.

> If those who are going to be doctors have no need of geometry, astronomy, dialectic, music or any other of the noble studies, as the most venerable Thessalus proclaimed, nor even of long experience and familiarity with the practice of the art, then it will be open to anyone to become a doctor without difficulty. That is why cobblers, carpenters, dyers and smiths rush into the practice of medicine. They abandon their previous trades, lay out their wares and vie for pride of place. For this reason I myself actually hesitated before writing on the method of healing – the method begun by the men of old (*palaioi*), which those who came after them attempted to complete. In the old days there was indeed great strife, as the men of Cos and Cnidus competed with each other simply in the number of their discoveries. These were the two families of Asclepiads in Asia, once that in Rhodes had fallen away; and the doctors from Italy, Philistion, Empedocles, Pausanias and their followers, strove with them too, the strife being of that fine kind, which was praised by Hesiod. There were, then, these three wonderful groups of doctors vying with each other. The Coan one prospered, and had the largest number of followers, as well as the best, followed closely by the Cnidian; but that from Italy one was also of great worth. None of those individuals went at sunrise to the houses of the rich to greet them, nor to dine with them in the evening, but, as Hesiod has it –
>
> > one who lacks work will look on another
> > as rich – the one who labours to plough and to plant
>
> – so too they constantly vied with each other, not to plough or plant the land, for these tasks would not be worthy of the race of the Asclepiads, though appropriate to the Ascraean poet, but to cultivate, continually increase and attempt to complete the art of Apollo and Asclepius.
>
> Now, however, that noble strife has ceased, or at least there remains only a small, faint remnant of it among humankind; it has been replaced by the wicked kind, and there is none who can mend it or heal it. As Hesiod says:

---

18 See note 30 below.

> Let not evil strife restrain your spirt from action.
>
> This is the sort of strife which – as again the poet Hesiod puts it –
>
> She raises her head, small at first, but later
> it stretches to heaven as she bestrides the earth.
>
> It is this strife that has driven Thessalus mad, so that he criticizes Hippocrates and the other Asclepiads, populating the wide theatre of the civilized world with his own books, then having himself judged within that theatre, winning the victory and being crowned over all the ancients, according to his own pronouncement.[19]

Three things are particularly worth noting here. One is the specific historical – and historically influential – view that Galen advances, whereby the schools of Cos and Cnidus, alongside the alternative views of Empedocles and Philistion, on the other side of Magna Graecia, represented the main strands in ancient medical thought. Secondly, we note that Galen's most rhetorically powerful elevation of the status of the ancients goes hand in hand with his most virulent attack on his arch-enemy, the leader of the Methodists, Thessalus. The two strands are inseparable: a key role of Galen's 'classicism' is precisely the refutation of rivals – above all, decadent, ill-educated, modern rivals. The third point to which I draw attention is the striking role taken by *competitiveness* in this passage. Central and recurrent in Galen's attack on contemporaries is their striving for status, their constant quarrelsome competitiveness. Here, in a neat reversal, *even competitiveness* was a positive thing in that distant, halcyon age.

Another aspect of the golden, pre-sectarian era, on Galen's account, is the preservation of knowledge within the family of the Asclepiads – the descendants of Asclepius – and the fact that such knowledge was handed down father to son. This, of course, takes us far from the present-day world of careerist sparring and self-publicizing – let alone the world in which an upstart cobbler or weaver could dare to aspire to the art of medicine.

So, in another text – and in the most strikingly ambitious historiographical move of all – Galen claims that the lack of writings on anatomy from that age is due, not to any lack of knowledge, but to the fact (arising precisely from that culture of successors within the medical family or guild) that such anatomical knowledge was so well known within that circle, and so securely transmitted within it, that no such writings were needed.

> I do not blame the ancients for not writing on anatomical procedures, any more than I blame Marinus for doing so. For the former, it was unnecessary to write such notes for themselves or for others, since they were trained from childhood by their parents to dissect,

---

[19] *The Therapeutic Method* 1.1 (X.5–7 K.)

as much as they were to read and write. The ancients – not just doctors, but also philosophers – had a serious engagement with the practice of anatomy. There was thus no fear that people who had learnt in this way would forget the manner of the procedures, any more than those who have practised the writing of letters from an early age would forget that. As time went on, however, it was decided to share the art not just with descendants, but with people outside the family ... once the childhood training was lost, it automatically followed that the learning deteriorated. ... It was after the art had ceased to be kept within the family of the Asclepiads, and had then become gradually worse through a series of such transmissions, that written materials were needed to ensure its preservation. ...[20]

This, then, is how Galen characterizes the gulf between the level of knowledge of the ancients and that of subsequent generations. There is a distinct peculiarity of the argumentative procedure arising from this self-positioning – a peculiarity which can escape our notice precisely because it becomes so familiar to us as we read texts of this period. Galen prefers to take as his imagined interlocutors, and to conduct his polemics in relation to, individuals who lived and wrote between 650 and 350 years ago, rather than his own contemporaries, or even authors of the previous generation or two.

I give just two examples. Much of *The Doctrines of Hippocrates and Plato* is taken up with an extended refutation of the views of Chrysippus, the Stoic philosopher of the third century BCE; and this polemic is conducted in an *ad hominem* manner, as if the author were present in the debate and able to answer for himself. Chrysippus' internal inconsistencies, the inadequacy of his fundamental psychological model to do justice to observed and experienced reality, the inappropriateness of the literary sources to which he appeals to establish this model, and even particular failures or missed opportunities within this last attempted project – all are exposed, on the basis of close and detailed examination and dissection of Chrysippus' own writings.

Aristotle – who, as observed above, is in many ways an authority figure for Galen, one of, though by no means the chief amongst, his venerated *palaioi*, and whose work is crucial to Galen's especially in the areas of logical method and element theory – is subjected to a similar, though less extended, polemic in the context of his views on embryology. Here, too, Galen detects internal inconsistency and absurdity in the relevant views; and here too he addresses his centuries-old opponent as though participating in a live debate with him.

This is not to say that Galen refuses to engage with authors and doctors of more recent times. On the contrary: some of his most direct and violent attacks, as we have already seen, are reserved for contemporaries or doctors of 'more re-

---

[20] *Anatomical Procedures* 2.1 (II.280–1 K.)

cent' times (*neōteroi*), most prominently the rival Methodist sect, which enjoyed considerable popularity in his time, and their leader Thessalus, who worked, and established the principles of this new sect, in the middle of the first century CE. Of course, this hostility to the modish new school, and his attempt to embarrass them through the authority of figures from the fifth and fourth century BCE, is itself a very obvious assertion of classicism on Galen's part. It seems clear, indeed, that one central part of the Methodists' appeal, connected with their mantra that 'the whole of the art of medicine can be taught within six months', was precisely their *rejection* of such classicizing knowledge. Their claim, in other words, was that medicine could be practised equally – in fact more – successfully without all the scholarly apparatus and years of training that Galen insists on. Theirs was an attractively minimalist theoretical model, making the claim to be able to deal with all clinical cases in practice, but *not* making the detailed knowledge claims made by a Galen about the internal composition and anatomy of the body – let alone the attendant knowledge of ancient authors and textual traditions. This rival school, then, not only enjoyed considerable success, in terms of its uptake by patients, but also in effect opened up the medical profession to a range of individuals of a very different level of education and from a very different background from Galen himself.

This situation raises an important question about the extent of ancient consensus on Hippocratic authority – a question to which it is difficult to give a precise answer. On the one hand, Galen's reverence for Hippocrates, and appeal to his authority, cannot be seen in isolation; it belongs closely, as already suggested, within the classicizing intellectual and literary culture of his time. In the more specific context of *medical* texts, meanwhile, rather than that of literary texts and authorities more broadly, there is clear evidence of other authors from Galen's own time, and the generations immediately before it, also appealing to the authority of Hippocrates, even while asserting very different views. Indeed, Galen's texts themselves, and the context and manner of citation of Hippocratic texts within them, also make clear that there are doctors with rival views who are, just as much as Galen is, claiming Hippocrates on their side in the assertion of those views.[21] On the other hand, the example of the Methodists – alongside other practitioners, also from time to time glimpsed in Galen's writings – makes it clear that such a consensus on the practical medical value of Hippocrates was very far from universal. Galen's Hippocratically based polemics, then, are conducted partly against others who also claim Hippocratic authority but (in his view) do so wrongly, partly against those who reject it altogether.

---

21 See Lloyd (1993); von Staden (1989), (1997), (2006), (2009); Leith (2021).

Let us return, though, to the question of the *neōteroi*. I stated above that Galen prefers to express and position himself through dialogue with authors of a distant past, but that he also engages from time to time with the *neōteroi*; and we then looked at the example of Thessalus and the Methodists. Yet the example is in a sense unrepresentative. There is, in general, a rather clear difference between the way in which Galen talks of *palaioi* and that in which he talks of *neōteroi*. The former are distinct, named figures – the most frequently named, as we already saw, being Hippocrates and Plato, but with a few others, also named, in second or third rank. When it comes to the *neōteroi*, the situation is different. These are – with, as suggested, a few notable exceptions – shady, *unnamed* figures. When it comes to doctors of more recent times who have got things wrong in one way or another, Galen very frequently prefers to express his criticisms of such individuals in an obscure, anonymized manner, e.g. 'some of the *neōteroi*').

In doing so, he typically contrasts their long-windedness, illogicality, inability to construct coherent arguments and tendency to sophistical reasoning with the honesty and argumentative strengths of the ancients – again, often without making clear who, specifically, the target of such attacks is.[22]

Recent scholarship on Galen has pointed to his *cultural* isolation at Rome – his self-identification as Greek, and self-insulation from things Roman or Latin.[23] We may, I suggest, speak equally of his *temporal* self-insulation – his sense of himself as belonging outside his own time, of conversing on an equal level with the greats of the classical Greek past, and by contrast embarrassed by, or attempting to obscure, any connection with or influence from his own or recent times – even though such influences were in some cases doubtless stronger.

Is it, then, that an author like Galen, positioning himself intellectually within centuries-old debates, and conducting discussions on a personal basis with figures from the classical Greek past, sees himself as *belonging to* that past – that he regards himself as in some sense belonging in that time? Or should one say,

---

22 Moreover, this is true even in some cases where Galen grudgingly *accepts* something from the *neōteroi*. For Galen is at times prepared to admit that some *neōteroi* they have got something right, or that a 'neologism' of theirs may be accepted into general use. In some such cases, indeed, it seems clear that he has in fact been strongly influenced by such *neōteroi* (even though it can, relatedly, be quite difficult to identify the individuals in question). One such example is the fourfold division of 'materials of health' into things taken, things done, things evacuated and things that come into contact with us from outside. Galen adopts this classification from 'the most respectable of the *neōteroi*' at *Health* 1.15, 36 Koch (VI.78 K.) and 5.10, 154–5 Koch (VI.358 K.). It seems that the distinction may derive from Galen's near contemporaries Antyllus and Herodotus, though he mentions neither by name; see Singer (forthcoming).
23 See Swain (1996); Mattern (2008): 49.

rather, that his self-positioning is *atemporal* in nature, that through his scholarship, understanding and classically inspired intellectual striving he has transcended time altogether – as, presumably, have those classical hero figures themselves? In theory, the latter seems the better interpretation; or perhaps one does not have to decide between the two perceptions: transcendence and a fixation upon the classics of the fifth and fourth centuries merge into one in this intellectual world-view (which is, of course, from our scholarly perspective, a world-view which belongs very clearly to a specific historical moment). It is instructive to consider Galen's own idealized representation of the arts and their practitioners, existing – outside time and space, one must imagine – in circles around the god Hermes:

> The other band is a band of fine men: the practitioners of the arts. They do not run, nor do they shout, nor fight each other. In their midst is the god, and about him they are all ranged in order, never leaving the place that he has assigned them. Those nearest the god, forming a circle about him, are geometers, mathematicians, philosophers, doctors, astronomers and scholars. After them the second band: painters, sculptors, teachers, carpenters, architects and stone-workers; and after them the third order: all the other arts ... Socrates is among them, and Homer and Hippocrates, as well as Plato and his lovers; these are people to be revered like gods, as they are the god's subjects and servants. The others too, though, without exception receive the god's attention.[24]

So, a broad picture has emerged of Galen's attitude to the past and, relatedly, four central features of his argumentative practice:

(a) he exalts the ancients over the moderns;
(b) he prefers to place his own views in relation to those of the former rather than those of the latter;
(c) he contrasts the sound argumentative practices and ethical motivations of the former with the vanity, competitiveness and sophistical confusions of the latter;
(d) he usually mentions the great *palaioi* clearly by name, while often referring to the *neōteroi* not just in disparaging, but also in vague and anonymizing, terms.

In this picture, then, we behold Galen the ideologue in his attitude to past and present time, and in his self-positioning within – or perhaps better, outside – it. It is a picture which reflects an undeniable, indeed absolutely central, aspect of his approach to the tradition and to his contemporaries.

---

24 *An Exhortation to Follow the Arts* 5, 118–20 Barigazzi (I.6–7 K.).

Galen on the old and the new (2): historiography and periodization

Yet there is another side to the story – and one which is of considerable interest for our enquiry, as it sheds light on the view ancient authors had of distinct periods within their own past, on the development of the historiographical practice of periodization. For, alongside the ideological and indeed idealizing version of history just considered, there is another, wherein Galen is much more pragmatic and neutral – and indeed precise and informative – in his historical accounts, and in which the 'old' and the 'new' appear as straightforwardly chronological, rather than morally loaded, terms.

So, for example, Galen does not always line up ancients against moderns in his accounts of previous authority; the 'line of authority' can cross the *palaioi* / *neōteroi* distinction, as when the frequently suspect recent doctor Athenaeus is lined up alongside his more usually respected, and earlier, authorities, or when that frequent butt of his polemic, Asclepiades, forms part of a near-universal consensus against Erasistratus.[25] Moreover, there are clear cases where he takes his terminology or distinctions from moderns rather than ancients, even though he obscures the extent of this, or, in some cases where he admits it, is unspecific about *who*, in the recent tradition, he is indebted to.[26]

There are also cases, especially in discussions of terminology, where references to the *neōteroi* are entirely neutral. It is not, in such cases, that they are being accused of obfuscation or confusion; it is simply that usage has changed since the times of Hippocrates, and we must be aware of this in order to avoid misunderstanding in our reading of those earlier texts. (An obvious example is the

---

25 In the former case, Athenaeus is claimed as part of the broad consensus on the nature of the composition of the human body from the four fundamental qualities, alongside Diocles, Mnesitheus, Dieuches, 'and practically all the best-reputed doctors ... and best philosophers' (καὶ σχέδον πᾶσι τοῖς εὐδοκιμωτάτοις ἰατροῖς ... καὶ τῶν φιλοσόφων τοῖς ἀρίστοις), *The Therapeutic Method* 7.3 (X.462 K.). In the latter, Asclepiades is brought on side in favour of the therapeutic value of venesection, *Venesection, against Erasistratus* 5 (XI.163 K.). In the latter passage, indeed, the fact that even the constantly quarrelsome Asclepiades, who 'rejects almost all previous views', and is implacably anti-Hippocratic, nevertheless supports venesection, and that people who agree on practically everything else agree on this, itself strengthens the argument. For, as he adds, 'I think nothing more worthy of trust than an agreement which involves no grounds for suspicion' (ἐμοὶ μὲν γὰρ οὐδὲν εἶναι δοκεῖ πιστότερον ἀνυπόπτου συμφωνίας).

26 See note 22 above. Further cases where he polemicizes against a recent author but in fact seems likely to be fundamentally indebted to him are those of Athenaeus, on whom see *Mixtures*, with the discussion of Singer and van der Eijk (2018) and, in pulse theory, Archigenes, on whom see von Staden (1991).

'more recent' usage, unproblematically adopted by Galen but as he admits unknown to Hippocrates, whereby arteries are referred to by the term *artēriai* and not, in a way undifferentiated from veins, as *phlebes*.) But we can go still further: there are in fact cases where the writings of the *neōteroi* are to be preferred to the those of the *palaioi:* this is because – in pharmacological writings, especially – a more recent writer will accumulate all the information from the earlier writers and add something of his own. In some cases, then, the writings of the *neōteroi* are simply better, more complete, or informed by further research or experience.[27] The sense of reverence for the ancients here sits – albeit perhaps rather awkwardly – alongside a notion of scientific progress which would be much more familiar to us today. But it is a notion which Galen explicitly accepts. Hippocrates made the best start, to be sure – and of course those moderns who ignore or criticize him are barking up the wrong tree – but you cannot expect the same person to start an art and to complete it. Here, there is a wholly legitimate and indeed necessary role for recent and contemporary authors in improving on and perfecting the ancient body of knowledge.[28]

The case of anatomy – touched on above – is of particular interest here. In spite of (or as Galen might optimistically claim, consistently with) his claim that Hippocrates had a high level of anatomical knowledge, which however was never consigned to the page, Galen himself gained his own anatomical knowledge from a much more recent tradition, that of the 'school of Quintus', a set of teachers and texts of anatomy of the immediately preceding generations.[29] Nor does Galen – if one looks in the right places in his work – deny his indebtedness to this recent school; indeed he emphasizes his desperation, as a young man, to find and study with its best contemporary representatives, implying that he saw this as the only way to acquire a sound training in anatomy. Moreover, he is quite clear about the timeline, explicitly placing Quintus in the reign of Hadrian, and attributing the revival of anatomical activity to Marinus, on whose treatises Galen himself wrote extensive commentaries, immediately be-

---

[27] *The Composition of Drugs according to Place* 2.1 (XII.501 K.) and 6.9 (XII.988–9 K.).
[28] Consider the remark in *The Best Doctor is Also a Philosopher* (3): 'It would be easy, for example, to learn thoroughly in a very few years what Hippocrates discovered over a very long period of time; and then to devote the rest of one's life to the discovery of what remains'. For this Galenic view of scientific progress see Hankinson (1994).
[29] See von Staden (1992); Grmek and Gourevitch (1994); Singer (2019a); Salas (2021); Salas (forthcoming).

fore that.³⁰ It is, however, noteworthy that, with the exception of Marinus himself, he does not *explicitly* refer to them as *neōteroi*, even though they clearly are so according to his own periodization.

Which leads us, finally, to the most striking aspect of this alternative analysis of Galen's historicizing remarks – the analysis in terms of straightforward chronology as opposed to ideological self-positioning. For in fact Galen, in his account of previous medical authors, is capable of being surprisingly precise in his positioning of them within historical periods. To be sure, there are no precise birth or death dates in this kind of historiography, nor – with a few exceptions – references to datable periods or moments, such as a regnal period or its end. The few such references that there are, however, combine with a number of remarks about relative period and influence, enabling us to see that Galen in fact has a pretty clear picture of the succession of authors previous to and up to his own time, understood in terms of fairly precise historical periods.

In fact – in spite of what has been said above about the fluid nature of both *palaioi* and *neōteroi* – Galen at one point gives an exact date for the division between the two eras – namely, that of the death of Alexander.³¹

It is worth digressing here for a moment to consider some other well-known ancient connotations of the term *neōteroi*. To the reader of ancient literary texts it is particularly well known as the term applied to the 'new poets' of the first century BCE at Rome, poets who probably included Catullus and who took their inspiration from more recent rather than 'classical' sources.³² Specifically, the sources of this inspiration were the Hellenistic poets, for example Callimachus and Theocritus, who belonged, precisely, to the period immediately after the death of Alexander. Callimachus was a prominent scholar at the Library of Alexandria; and it is from this milieu – a milieu in which Galen too had studied, albeit several centuries later – that the scholarly distinction between *neōteroi* and *palaioi* itself arises.

---

30 See *Anatomical Procedures* 14.1, 167 Simon; at *The Doctrines of Hippocrates and Plato* 8.1, 480 De Lacy (V.650 K.) Marinus is characterized as 'the one who after the ancients restored anatomy, which had been neglected in the intervening time'.

31 See *Commentary on Hippocrates' Epidemics, book 6* 7, 399,10–11 Wenkebach/Pfaff, where he clarifies: 'by "more recent doctors" I mean all those who lived after the death of Alexander.' He mentions the death of Alexander as a temporal demarcator also at *Commentary on the Nature of the Human Being* 1.44, 55,10–14 Mewaldt (XV.105 K.).

32 Cicero uses both the Greek term *neōteroi* and the Latin *poetae novi* to refer to some poets of his time (*Letters to Atticus* 7.2.1; *The Orator* 161 (cf. 168 on 'antiqui')); there is some debate as to how precise a group he has in mind with these designations, and indeed whether Catullus is included.

Now, of course, it may be argued that this one particular gloss on the sense of the term *neōteroi*, appearing at one particular point in Galen's extant work, should not be given excessive weight – even if it does, undoubtedly, provide a point of curiosity that the single precise criterion of periodization that Galen mentions – that of the death of Alexander – is one still used in historiographical periodizations today. Certainly, we must not expect that Galen elsewhere follows that specification with complete consistency; and indeed it would be wrong to look for absolute precision in the reference of a term – a comparative adjective, to boot – which, as we have already observed, is used in a variety of argumentative contexts, often with disparaging rhetorical force.

Nonetheless, by placing this remark alongside the others in which Galen refers to previous sources using the terminology of *palaios* or *neōteros*, a pretty consistent picture emerges, not just of the identity of those individuals who fall within the domain of each adjective, but also of their chronological relationship in more detail. In the following table, not every author mentioned by Galen has been included; the intention rather has been to include all those mentioned in the context of the use of the terms *palaios* and *neōteros*, and thus to clarify his understanding of historical periods as it emerges through the use of this classification.[33]

TABLE 7: Galen's periodization of the past

Broad designation or period	Further chronological divisions	Doctors	Notes on doctors	Philosophers
palaioi	Hippocratic period	Hippocrates and contemporaries: Euryphon, Philistion, Ariston, Pherecydes, Polybus	some of these actually pre-Hippocratic: *Commentary on Hippocrates' Regimen in Acute Diseases* 1.17, 134–5; cf. *Commentary on Hippocrates' Aphorisms* 1	Plato, Aristotle, Theophrastus

---

[33] It will be observed that the table is skimpy in the information given about philosophers, as opposed to doctors. Here Galen mentions fewer individuals, and perhaps operates with a less clear sense of relative date. In any case, I have not attempted, in this last column, to do justice to the chronological picture Galen may have in mind, e. g. as relates to Chrysippus and Posidonius; it seemed worthwhile, nevertheless, to include this last column, as there are a few very chronologically clear cases whom Galen does mention in this category.

TABLE 7: Galen's periodization of the past *(Continued)*

Broad designation or period	Further chronological divisions	Doctors	Notes on doctors	Philosophers
palaioi	earlier 'ancients'	[after Hippocrates, earlier period:] Diocles (4th), Praxagoras (4th) Pleistonicus (4th/3rd), Mnesitheus (4th), Dieuches (4th)	Most are mentioned without further specification, but seem to belong to earlier period by contrast with those in the following group	
	later 'ancients'	Philotimus, Eudemus, Herophilus	Classed as *palaioi*, but also as contemporaries of Erasistratus, by contrast with e.g. Diocles, Praxagoras; cf. *The Therapeutic Method* 1.3 (X.28 K.), where Philotimus and Herophilus are co-students and Praxagoras teacher of the former (or of Herophilus?)	
around the death of Alexander		Erasistratus	Classed as *palaios*, e.g. *Simple Drugs* 1.29 (XI.433 K.); often listed alongside *neōteroi* though not explicitly *neōteros*	
neōteroi	earlier *neōteroi*	Asclepiades; Athenaeus		Favorinus; *neōteroi* Stoics are mentioned at VII.527 K.
	later *neōteroi*	Archigenes, Agathinus, Marinus, [Quintus], Rufus, Sabinus	Archigenes and Agathinus particularly late *neōteroi*; Marinus in century before Galen	
	contemporaries	the Erasistrateans and Methodists at Rome		

A few points – some of them summarized in the fourth column of the table – are particularly worthy of note. One is that Galen has a fairly clear conception of a Hippocratic age: in discussion of the linguistic usage of that period, as well as of the possible attribution of 'Hippocratic' works to other authors of a similar age, Philistion, Ariston, Euryphon and Pherecydes and Polybus emerge clearly as the relevant set of individuals – some direct contemporaries of the great man, some a little earlier or later. Then, we find later subdivisions, still *within* the period covered by the term *palaioi*. Diocles and Praxagoras consistently appear in lists of authorities as closely following Hippocrates; moreover, they are explicitly mentioned as belonging to an earlier phase than Philotimus, Herophilus and Eudemus, even though the latter are still *palaioi*.

There seem to be divisions within the age of the *neōteroi*, too. Of course, as observed already, the term can cover a broad range, and can even include Galen's actual, unnamed, contemporaries – the Erasistrateans or Methodists currently practising in Rome. And the fixing of the starting-point of the era at the death of Alexander only adds to this sense: this is a span of more than 500 years to Galen's own time. Still, there are further implied subdivisions; when Galen uses a phrase like 'the *neōteroi* who came after him [sc. Erasistratus] right up to the followers or Archigenes',[34] it seems that he means to place Archigenes and his followers in the most recent phase. And, as we have seen, Galen is explicit about placing Quintus (though he does not explicitly refer to him as a *neōteros*), in the reign of Hadrian, with Marinus a little older than him. Asclepiades, and probably Athenaeus, belong to a stage quite a bit earlier than that.

Most striking of all is the position of Erasistratus, who seems to be on the edge of the two periods; at least once he is referred to as *palaios*; at other times, while not explicitly placed in the category of *neōteroi*, he is mentioned alongside them. It is tempting to say that this liminal position reflects Galen's ambivalent attitude to him: in some contexts a respected anatomical authority, to whom Galen seems clearly indebted in aspects of his own physiological theory, especially in the area of the nervous system, he is severely criticized for his inadequate account of physiological motions in the body, as well as for his outright rejection of venesection in all clinical cases. Now that we have gained some clarity about the nature of Galen's chronological periodization, however, we might see Erasistratus' liminal position rather as a function of that: his birth date was – according to modern scholarship at least – very close to that watershed of the death of Alexander; he was, probably, the first of the authors in the above table to be born after it.

---

[34] *Commentary on Hippocrates' Aphorisms* 1 (XVIIIA.7 K.). This passage, which is about the views of Erasistratus, mentions Philotimus, Eudemus and Herophilus as roughly contemporary with him, as distinct from a group of earlier doctors, such as Diocles.

Thus, in spite of the strong ideological, nostalgic and idealizing account of the past, and the use of the terms *palaios* and *neōteros* within that account, we also see the parallel development within Galen of a strikingly 'modern' conception of distinct historical periods and their relationship.

Galen on his own age

What, then, of Galen's own period: does this acquire a particular definition or status? As we have seen already in his nostalgia for a 'golden age', he regards his own as decadent. Most of his remarks along these lines – taking us back to the culturally embedded perception of a distant golden age from which our own represents a disastrous decline – do not depart greatly from the moralizing clichés that one encounters in many a literary text, texts of satire for example.[35] The main context of it, in Galen, is somewhat more specific than that: it is *intellectual* vanity or fraudulence and unethical behaviour in specifically *medical* contexts that exercise him particularly.

The extended quotation from *The Therapeutic Method* above gave a flavour of the recurrent rhetoric. The central points of this rhetoric recur in treatise after treatise (and in most concentrated form in *Affections and Errors*, in the *Exhortation* and in *The Best Doctor is Also a Philosopher*). People of today are more interested in money and reputation than in the arts in general, medicine in particular; they therefore attend on and flatter the rich to the detriment of both their characters and their practice of the art; intellectual and medical life is dominated by sectarian competitiveness, and by practitioners whose poor training in logic, or addiction to sophistical argument, lead them into fatal error.

The positive ethical aspirations, for a truly philanthropic and disinterested doctor or intellectual, are summarized as follows (with plenty of reference to their contrasted opposites):

> So, the person who wishes to attain to such a character will, necessarily, not only despise money, but also be extremely hardworking. And one cannot be hardworking if one is continually drinking or eating or indulging in sex: if, to put it briefly, one is a slave to genitals and belly. The true doctor has been found to be a lover of Self-restraint and a follower of Truth. Furthermore, he must train himself in logical method to know how many diseases there are, by species and by genus, and how, in each case, one is to discover an indication of the treatment. This same method also provides the foundations for knowledge of the

---

35 On Galen's own relationship to the literary satire tradition, see Rosen (2010).

body's very nature ... He must, therefore, possess all the parts of philosophy: the logical, the physical and the ethical.[36]

The partially autobiographical text *Prognosis* elaborates the picture of a society, medical society in particular, riven with rivalry and backstabbing, and adds the further accusation that fraudulent doctors who strive for success in society are driven by their ambition and jealousy to conspire against any genuine practitioner who comes along, slandering him, hounding him out of the city, or worse.[37]

There is nothing here, of course, which is in any way specific to one particular period: the sense is a general one of ethical and intellectual decline – even though this sense is backed up by some extraordinarily vivid accounts of individual instances of rivalry and public confrontation, as well as of stupidity and intellectual incompetence. Again, none of this takes us very far from standard literary tropes of present-day corruption and decline, familiar from many another moralizing or satirical author.

Nor is there any sense, to counteract this, that Galen might – in spite of his close association with the emperor Marcus Aurelius, and *pace* Edward Gibbon – have discerned any positive aspect in the 'spirit of his age', that he might have thought of it as especially peaceful, prosperous, or well managed. Positive or negative remarks concerning the characters and behaviour of individual emperors (and other members of the imperial family) there are, but these remain just that: characterizations of a particular individual or of his or her effects on those around them, not in any sense broader reflections on the spirit of an age. It is not just that Galen has nothing elevated (on Gibbonian or other lines) to say about the age, considered in such political or cultural terms; he does not evince a negative or problematized account of it, in such terms, either. (One might think here of Dodds' 'age of anxiety', or indeed more broadly of historical analyses which detect a cultural transition at this point, shifts or uncertainties related to the rise of Christianity, for example.)[38] Simply, any such a perspective is absent from his writings. An arguable exception is his account of the reign of Commodus, which, certainly, Galen characterizes as a reign of terror; but here, again, we are talking about his discussion of an individual tyrant and his behaviour, not any view of the age in a broader or more abstract sense. As for Galen's attitude to Roman sovereignty, to the *pax Romana* in general, the most we can say, I think, is that he takes it as a fact of life, to be acknowledged and worked with

---

36 *The Best Doctor is Also a Philosopher* 2–3.
37 See especially *Prognosis* 1, 68–74 Nutton (XIV.601–4 K.), mentioning the case of Quintus, who was apparently expelled from Rome on a charge of having murdered his patients.
38 Dodds (1965).

for practical purposes. If he makes an occasional remark, for example, about the extent of Roman rule, or about such-and-such a drug being imported from outside the *oikoumenē*, he seems to be speaking in purely factual or practical terms, to delineate actual geographical boundaries.[39] No sense arises from his work, either that things are well or badly governed on this dispensation or, indeed that things could be in any way imagined differently.

Again, we have the sense of an author culturally and mentally detached from his actual place and time – a time, indeed, that he is not concerned to delineate or characterize with any detail, other than the kind of detail provided by a range of standard moralizing clichés.

Galen on his own life and works

So, Galen appears in his own work as in a sense transcending his times – his oeuvre and his life's project existing in a classical Greek, perhaps better an atemporal realm, in which he hobnobs with the likes of Hippocrates – rather as he does, indeed, in many a later visual portrayal of him.

Yet, for all that, Galen is one of the most anecdotal and specific writers of antiquity, in the details he gives us of everyday, literary and intellectual life; and this applies too to his own autobiography. His two accounts of his own writings, indeed (which have been dubbed works of 'auto-bibliography') are – alongside the recently discovered account of his losses in the great fire of 192 CE, *Avoiding Distress* – amongst the most fascinating documents of the period, from the point of view of ancient biography and from that of ancient book culture.[40]

---

39 His remarks, considered in the previous chapter, about the prevalence of famine in rural areas 'amongst many of the peoples who are subject to Roman rule' (see 62–3 with nn. 53–4) could be read as critical of the economic and political status quo, but any such criticism is certainly not the point of those remarks, nor something made explicit. Other similar references to Roman rule seem straightforwardly neutral, intended simply to clarify points of nomenclature or translation, for example a reference to *silingnitis* and *semidalis* as the words used, 'by the Romans and almost all those over whom they rule', for the purest form of wheat or bread (*The Capacities of Foodstuffs* 1.2, 218 Helmreich, VI.483 K.), or another to the different measures in use 'before Roman power had been so widely extended' (*The Composition of Drugs according to Kind* 1.15, XIII.428–9 K.).
40 For analysis of what these texts tell us not only about Galen's own practices, but about scholarship, libraries, book composition and book distribution in the ancient world more generally, see Singer (2019b).

There is, I think, a tension here – a tension between two different ways of chronicling or analysing one's own work, and in the same process, of telling one's own life story. On the one hand, the account is tied to individual, contingent datable events; on the other, what is being presented is not a narrative, but a curriculum, an order of instruction – an ideally interlocking system, in which the important thing is not the chronological order of the texts' composition, but the fact that they permanently co-exist, in a perfect, perfectly cross-referrable, corpus.

The tension strikes us if we simply look at the series of chapter headings in *My Own Books*. Such titles as 'works written during my first stay in Rome', and the even more precise and contingent 'books of my own composition which were given to me by certain parties on my return home', sit alongside such titles as those of ch. 4, 'works of anatomical science', ch. 5, 'books containing the activities and functions of the parts made apparent in anatomy', ch. 6, 'necessary study preliminary to the method of healing', ch. 7, 'works of therapeutics', ch. 8: 'works of prognostic science'. There is then a whole range of other such thematic chapter headings, including specific topics in philosophy (ch. 14: demonstration; ch. 15: ethics) and individual philosophical and medical authors (the Stoics, Epicurus, Erasistratus, Asclepiades). But those just cited, chapter headings 4–8, are particularly worthy of our attention. They indicate the way in which Galen organizes his works in an ideal paedagogic order, or order of instruction. For the student, the study of anatomy underlies that of physiology ('activities and functions of the parts'), from which in turn one proceeds to the study 'preliminary to the method of healing' (which is, essentially, that of the physical composition of the body and the pathological changes that take place within it, thus including disease classification). From this one proceeds to the study of therapeutics proper, and so to prognosis (which focuses centrally on the study of the pulse and on that of crises and critical days, which we will revisit at some length in the next chapter).

As already indicated, this thematic organization of the corpus is not consistently followed. There is the partial chronological ordering of works already mentioned, especially in the early chapters of *My Own Books*; and the account of the Hippocratic commentaries in ch. 9, immediately following the 'curriculum' chapters (4–8) just summarized, digresses into an account of the original purpose, justification and intended readerships of the works in question, as well as the chronological order of their composition. And the rationale of composition, and in some cases of rewriting, of certain works is explained in terms of an original public argumentative context or of the original intended addressee, or sometimes the premature departure of this addressee. There are, moreover, a few actual titles of (lost) works which are tied to particular, more or less datable, events, although these are very much the exceptions.[41]

It should be noted, too, though the point cannot be explored here in detail, that there is a further tension: that between Galen's sense of the validity and solidity of his corpus as a paedagogic resource, and the repeated claims that he originally intended nothing for public distribution, that his works were distributed against his better judgement, and often written, again reluctantly, at the behest of friends or students.[42]

There is, then, some toing and froing between a chronological and contingent account and a thematic one. But the thematic one dominates; and, more than that, the notion of an ideal order of medical instruction, of which Galen's own works are the ideal instantiation, is central to Galen's view of his works, far beyond the account given in *My Own Books*. There is, indeed, a work specifically entitled *The Order of My Own Books*, which again presents his works as constituting such a curriculum (although, in fact, *My Own Books* in several ways presents a clearer and fuller picture of this). But beyond these works of auto-bibliography, and indeed permeating his writings quite generally, we find a wealth of forward and backward references, which betoken the same fundamental Galenic sense of a stable and abiding corpus of his own works.

It will be worth our while to consider these cross-references in a bit more detail. What does it mean when an ancient author says, 'as we shall discuss in work X', or 'as was stated in work Y'? The obvious interpretation, from a modern perspective, might be a straightforward chronological one: work X has not yet been written, while work Y has. But this obvious interpretation may hide a more complex reality. Texts in the ancient world were, to a large extent, orally composed; technical medical treatises in particular may have an original context of oral instruction, of which the text which we have now is the written record or final version; texts could exist in a provisional form, distributed perhaps to a smaller inner circle, before reaching the stage of final 'publication' (itself not a straightforward concept in Graeco-Roman culture). Galen in fact gives us detailed evidence of all these processes, in the context of his own work.

---

41 Most notably, 'things said in public in the time of Pertinax', where, without further information, both the nature of the things said and the rationale for placing them under this particular heading must remain matters of speculation. Such a title as 'the discourse with Bacchides and Cyrus in the villa of Menarchus' is also one tied to a datable event, albeit only datable, presumably, to those in a small circle of acquaintances.
42 For analysis of Galen's self-presentation of his life and works, and of this apparently contradictory position, see Boudon-Millot (2009); Vegetti (2013): 31–52.

A forward reference to another text, of the form just mentioned, *could* also be taken as a reference to an existing work: it could be saying, in effect: we shall discuss this when we get to that point in the lecture course. At the very least, it indicates the existence of the work in outline, in planned form. Some of Galen's cross-references are ambiguous as to whether they indicate a particular work in which something has already been written, or rather define a separate subject area, the fact that this belongs to a different discussion. And, certainly – something that has provided a headache to those scholars who have struggled through this thorny terrain – the *chronological* picture arising from the totality of backward and forward cross-references is not a consistent one. Close analysis of all such references will lead to the conclusion that the same work is situated both in the past and in the future, with respect to a particular other work. The picture that emerges is, at the very least, one of texts existing in provisional form, and liable to constant updating (such cross-references can, of course, easily be added in the process of fairly superficial revision). One might, more strongly, be tempted to say that chronological future and past are not what are centrally at issue in such references; rather, these are a set of internal cross-references to a body of work conceived as existing trans-temporally.

And yet, linear biography is important too. Both in *My Own Books* and elsewhere, most notably in *Prognosis, Affections and Errors of the Soul* and – in relation to his anatomical education – *Anatomical Procedures*, Galen outlines the crucial moments and phases of his early education, in both philosophy and medicine. In his conception of his own biography, those developmental phases are essential in order, in a sense, to justify what follows. And there is a point to be considered here, perhaps also of wider interest for the construction of ancient biographies, and certainly of potential relevance to our discussion in the previous chapter of the conceptual division of life spans. For – whether by chance or not – at least two of the moments that Galen identifies as crucial turning-points in his own development coincide with ends of hebdomads.

It is on the completion of his fourteenth year, Galen says, that he 'began to attend the lectures of philosophers of my home city'.[43] That may indeed – as indicated by our previous discussion – be the normal age at which such 'secondary', or more specialized, school education would be expected to begin; in any case, it is one of the few actual chronological ages that Galen mentions in relation to his own biography. If we move, then, to the end of the fourth hebdomad, the completion of his 28th year, we already noted, in the previous chapter, that Galen marks this out as a turning-point in terms of his own personal health. But

---

43 *Affections and Errors* 1.8, 28 De Boer (V.41 K.).

it coincides with a turning-point in his career, too. At the end of his 28th year, Galen had just finished a study tour, to Smyrna, Corinth and Alexandria, during which he acquired the basics of his anatomical and medical knowledge. At this point he returned to his home town and received his first appointment, as official doctor to the gladiators. The coincidence between the date of this appointment and the turning-point in his health has been noted in previous scholarship.[44] For it is not just his adoption of a more appropriate health regime that Galen dates to this moment; it is also a dramatic intervention by his patron god, Asclepius, who saved him from a potentially fatal abscess.[45]

What has not been noted, however, is the coincidence between *both* these events – the completion of studies and commencement of career, on the one hand, and the divine intervention and transformation of health, on the other – with that precise hebdomadic moment, the end of his 28th year.

Other transitions and developments in Galen's life, on his own account, are in general not linked with precise ages or dates, and where they are, the significance is less obvious than that of the ages considered above. It is, however, worth noting a couple of events which Galen does tie to a particular age. Galen dates his return to Rome to the end of his 37th year. That is simply a contingent date, of no theoretical significance; but it is important to note what is being emphasized here. Galen has reached the age of maturity; the context of his mention of his 37th year is the reference to – and implied apology for – a number of works written *before* that, at a much earlier date, by implication at an age of immaturity. Even more specifically, he connects the limitations of a particular work with the fact that he was 'still quite young, in my 34th year', when he wrote it. It may be an overreading to insist on the hebdomadic date of 35 as in some way implied here, between Galen's period of still imperfectly educated adulthood and that of his full intellectual maturity. But certainly some such boundary is being drawn between works produced at the earlier periods, before the beginning of his second stay at Rome, and those which follow.

And – in a way related to both that point and one considered in the previous chapter, namely the greater vagueness that inevitably attends the division of lifespans in their *later*, as opposed to *earlier* phases – when we move into later phases of Galen's life and literary output, there are no such clear markers or watershed moments. What we know of the relative date of Galen's works – those earlier ones aside – is what can be deduced on the (problematic, as already dis-

---

44 Pietrobelli (2013): 117.
45 *My Own Books* 3, 142 Boudon-Millot (XIX.18–19 K.); cf. *Bloodletting against Erasistratus* 4 (XI.314–15 K.).

cussed) basis of cross-references, on the one hand, and on that of very occasional references to datable or roughly datable events – Marcus Aurelius' absence from Rome (169–76), the fire in the Roman forum (192), the Antonine plague (much less definite) – on the other. The entire period from his late thirties onward, is presented, in an undifferentiated way, as that of his intellectual and medical maturity.

And this is the period of the vast majority of his writings. There is a point of importance to be considered here – a crucial point of difference, indeed, between this ancient approach to literary or intellectual biography and those which tend to dominate in modern scholarship. For what is *not* present, either explicitly or by implication, in Galen's autobiography or auto-bibliography is a *developmental* account of his works. Modern scholarship is constantly exercised to produce such accounts, to find internal, and where possible external, justification for it in the works of an author. Galenic scholarship has been far from immune from the tendency. And such development accounts are remarkably resistant to counter-arguments or methodological criticisms pointing to either the poverty of evidence supporting them or the strong risk of circularity that they run.[46]

Of course, it is open to modern scholars to argue for such developmental differences within the work of an author, if and when they find plausible evidence for it. Apart from the contingent fact, however, that the overwhelming majority of Galen's works were written after the age of 40, we should also consider, as it were, the more methodological or ideological consideration: such a developmental analysis is foreign to the perceptions of the ancient literary or intellectual biography itself. Apart from the few half-apologies for slightly immature works of his youth, already mentioned, Galen very rarely gives an example of a scientific or philosophical question on which he has actually changed his mind.[47] Otherwise, there is nothing that suggests that the body of work should be understood – at least in Galen's own self-conception – other than as a coherent system. In

---

[46] One thinks here of the methodological problems that attend developmental accounts of Plato's work. In the case of Galen, a strong developmental account was first advanced by Moraux (1984), focussing on *The Soul's Dependence on the Body* as the late culmination of his philosophical thought on the soul. Although, as I have argued elsewhere (2013), internal evidence of a significant difference in position between this work and others is at least highly questionable, and external evidence of its extreme lateness in Galen's output is non-existent, the view of this text as 'late', or even as written towards the end of Galen's life, has become firmly lodged in modern scholarship.

[47] Such a case – perhaps unique – is his account, in *The Shaping of the Embryo* (3, 66 Nickel, IV.663–4 K.) of his change of view on the order of formation of organs in the embryo since he wrote his earlier work, *Semen*.

terms of the planning and conceptualization of later work, equally, there is nothing that suggests the notion of a career path involving fundamental differences in direction or intellectual emphasis or interest over time.[48]

Let me add, as a coda, a final consideration of some relevance to both the questions just considered, that of the chronological vagueness of Galen's autobiographical remarks about his own later life, and that of the possibility or not of dating his works sequentially. This final consideration concerns the plague, already touched on the previous chapter. On the one hand, we saw how his references to it are strikingly imprecise and open-ended (above, pp. 61–2): we have the sense of an ongoing event, or one which even if concluded had no clear or recorded moment of its ending. Such writing seems, in a way, of a piece with what has been said above about the absence of clear defining moments in Galen's later, as opposed to his earlier and formative, life. If the plague has definitively come to an end in Galen's lifetime, he does not mention that, nor regard that ending as a moment of significance or watershed in his own later life – let alone give us some other identifiable external event, by which that moment could be fixed.

It is rather paradoxical, then, that the plague has sometimes been claimed in previous scholarship as just such a watershed, to be used to assist in the dating of Galen's works, since it is, in fact, one of the few events external to his own life and medical practice that Galen *does* mention. That is: by using the traditional end date of the Antonine plague in 180 CE, in conjunction with Galen's few references to it as current or recent, scholars hoped to provide an approximate date, or more often a *terminus post quem*, for the works in which those references occur.[49] Since, however, those references themselves are in several cases vague in their temporality, their 'now' indeterminate between present and recent past, and since, moreover, modern scholarship has moved away from that

---

48 Of course, that is not to say that Galen has no concept of *finding more time* for particular projects at different times, nor indeed to say that a different focus or range of intellectual interests may arise from the concentration on such projects. In this context, we may – albeit speculatively – point to the ethical works, and also much of the pharmacological work, and perhaps some of the Hippocratic commentaries, as being a late-life project, for which time was found after the completion of the works of core curriculum, and perhaps even after retirement. (Relevant here is Galen's remark that he will complete his project of Hippocratic commentary writing, 'if I live', *The Order of My Own Books* 3, 98 Boudon-Millot (XIX.57 K.), although the date of this remark is not certain.) It should, however, be emphasized that such a periodization *is* indeed speculative, and that the crucial difference between these works and those of the core curriculum remains precisely that – the thematic or conceptual one.
49 See Bardong (1942), drawing on the earlier work of J. Ilberg.

clear end date of 180, such use of the plague as a clear demarcator for biographical or bibliographical purposes seems doomed.[50]

We are left, then, with the former perception, that Galen's writing about the plague contributes to the unstructured, open-ended nature of his chronicling of the events of his mature life, largely devoid of clear markers or turning-points.

A parallel biography: Porphyry's *Life of Plotinus*

Our focus in this account of ancient intellectual bio-bibliography has been on Galen. This has been determined partly by reasons of space, and partly by the paucity of other closely parallel accounts – accounts, that is, from a similar period, which also discuss an intellectual's life history, and literary output, in detail. One such parallel, however, does suggest itself – that of Porphyry's *Life of Plotinus*, and it may be worth pointing to some analogies and disanalogies.

Of course, further such analogies could be made with a range of other biographical writings of the imperial period; any such broad survey is beyond my scope here. One thinks in particular of Plutarch's parallel-lives project, which is at once chronologically contingent and trans-temporal in its nature. It is hoped, however, that the case study here offered of Galenic autobiography, in conjunction with the parallel case of Porphyry, highlights some significant trends, and may be suggestive for future directions.[51]

Here, too, I shall argue, we find a tension between a contingent historiography, on the one hand, which ties the events and the writings of the subject's life to particular events, encounters and regnal periods, as well as providing contextual details of the original circumstances and peculiar context of a work's composition, preparation, or circulation, and a transtemporal one, on the other hand, considering the literary outcome of these contingent events and encounters as a solid and thematically interlocking corpus, communicating beyond its own time and, indeed, of eternal value.

---

50 On both the chronology of the plague and Galen's references to it, see Flemming (2019), who remarks that 'outbreaks certainly continued ... for decades thereafter' [sc., after the outbreaks of the 160s], and that the plague remains 'a feature of his writing at least into the 190s' (224).
51 Temporal attitudes in a range of ancient authors are explored in de Jong and Nünlist (2007). In his account of Philostratus' temporal narratives, Whitmarsh (2007) also suggests a fundamental dichotomy, namely one between 'regular' and 'paradigmatic' time (the former strictly chronological, the latter isolating especially important events). Such a dichotomy, while distinct from that which I suggest here in my analysis of Galen and Porphyry, perhaps functions in a somewhat parallel manner in the organization of and approach to events.

We may also point to some other common features of the ancient biographical project, especially in the way that divine favour intrudes into the narratives – albeit in very different contexts in the two cases – again in a sense taking us beyond normal time. Just as Asclepius' intervention shows his favour to the subject in Galen's own account of his early life, in the context of a delivery from death, so divine favour is shown to Plotinus by (among other things) the sudden appearance and disappearance of a snake, which by contrast indicates his auspicious delivery *to* death. (There is of course a disanalogy here too, both because the narration of a life by a disciple gives much greater scope for hagiography, and because Plotinus is in the nature of his perceived philosophical persona closer to the divine and a more likely subject for such theologically-based incidents.)

We encounter some difficulties at the outset. Plotinus himself is presented as, for philosophical reasons, resistant to the discussion of his own biography, especially details of birth and early life, including his precise birthday and birth date. (As if to counteract this reluctance, Porphyry seems exercised to produce a series of precise dates for moments in the master's life – his birth, his settling in Rome, his first writings.) Moreover, Plotinus, as a profoundly *atypical* student of philosophy, and, more generally, exemplar of Greek culture, bypasses the normal earlier developmental stages, and is certainly not undertaking philosophical studies at the age of 14; it seems dubious, too, whether any particular significance is to be attached to the specification of the 28th year as that in which Porphyry says that he *did* first turn to philosophy.

There are, I would suggest, just two main parallels between the presentation of Plotinus by Porphyry and Galen's self-presentation; but they are significant. First, Plotinus – even more so than Galen – goes through a variety of life experiences, travels and studies, and has reached late adulthood, before he writes anything. This is a biographical world where maturity is valued; there is no role for precocious genius. Secondly, and relatedly, his reluctance to write, the sense that he has to be persuaded to do so in some ways against his better judgement, is emphasized – emphasized by Porphyry in his account of Plotinus even more strongly than it is by Galen in his own case. The reasons for the reluctance are somewhat different within the two biographies, but there is a connection in both cases to the risks attendant on sending one's thoughts or writings into the world to be distorted and misunderstood.

Most crucially, Plotinus writes – or rather dictates – nothing before the age of maturity, and there is little sense that one should look for an internal development to the writings. Porphyry recounts that Plotinus moved to Rome at the age of forty, after his years of study with Ammonius and his expedition eastwards in the army of the emperor Gordian, and that for ten years he lectured and communicated within a small circle while writing nothing. He thus wrote his first essays around the age of 50; but even when Porphyry arrived nine years later, he had only written the first 21.

When it comes to the account of those writings themselves, it is indeed interesting to compare the interplay of chronological and thematic considerations here with that found in Galen. At their first mention in the *Life* (4–6), Porphyry lays out the writings chronologically, adding such attendant background considerations as Porphyry's presence or absence at the time, and the ruling emperor; again we get, as with Galen, a sense of the occasional and context-specific nature of their original composition. Yet, as is well known, Porphyry had the responsibility for the edition of Plotinus' works, whereby he organized them, on thematic lines, into the 'Enneads' known to us today, in a way which obscures both relative chronology and original context. And there is no suggestion in the *Life* that such a chronology should be regarded as significant *for philosophical content*. Porphyry does, however, make a division into three phases, which differ in terms rather of *strength of capacity* – according to whether Plotinus was in his early manhood, his vigorous prime, or a state of bodily decline. The first essays were written 'in his first life stage (*hēlikia*)', the second, main set when he was 'in his prime', the last when he was 'worn down by his body' (6).

The mention of the 'first life stage' and 'prime' here are striking, and take us back to the discussion of the previous chapter. Yet we observe that their appearance here cannot correspond to any normal understanding of human biology. No traditional, let alone medical, division of life stages of the sort that we have considered would have a man entering the prime at the age of 59; and the terminology of 'first life stage' for the ten years before that is also, in normal terms, bizarre. What we seem to have is a philosophically specific – perhaps even Plotinus-specific – notion of the age of maturity. It is, however, possible to relate it to a remark Galen makes, about the psychic powers continuing or increasing in excellence at a later period, while the physical ones are in decline (see above, p. 50 with n. 35). The last few years of Plotinus' life, however, are considered ones of a partial intellectual deterioration.

But in spite of this acknowledgement of a bodily and intellectual increase and diminution in energy, what is emphasized, again, is the maturity acquired *before* the writing project, on the one hand, and the coherence, the fundamentally atemporal nature, of the written work, on the other.

The tension between a chronological account, beset with contingent details of emperors, students, personal events and encounters, and physical challenges, and the atemporal solidity – the eternal validity – of the corpus, runs through the two works, Galen's autobiography and Plotinus' biography, in different ways. In both, atemporality dominates – albeit an atemporality with the counterpoint of a series of interfering, contingent events. Both manifest certain features of the conception and patterning of an intellectual's life which are strikingly different from their modern counterparts.

Chapter Four:
Time for the doctor: crises, perils and opportunities

In the second chapter we considered two cycles of fundamental importance for the perception and management of time: the cycle of life and the cycle of the seasons. In this chapter we shall look at another cycle of equal potential importance – the monthly one. While making no attempt to consider this cycle in general terms, or to do justice its full significance in a range of areas (for example, the gynaecological or the astrological), we shall explore one particular significance the monthly cycle acquired in ancient medical theory and practice, in relation to the diagnosis and treatment of fevers. In the process, we shall also be exploring concepts which were central to the medical discourse and remained influential for centuries – those of the crisis (*krisis*), the critical day or hour and the *kairos*.

Kairos, *krisis* and *peira*: a perilous time

Everyone – even one completely ignorant of the conceptual world of Graeco-Roman medicine – knows that life is short; and someone with even the most cursory knowledge of it will also be aware that the art is long. The Hippocratic aphorism – the very first one of all – which begins with those words of wisdom continues with the following:

> the *kairos* is fleeting, the *krisis* dangerous, *peira* precarious[1]

These three phrases, in which I have left the nouns untranslated, in fact summarize in a few pithy words the terrifying maze of perils, challenges and complexities presented by the world of Graeco-Roman clinical medicine – the world into which we shall now venture.

Kairos may most accurately, if not most elegantly, be translated 'right time' or 'opportune moment'. The notion was to become central to the doctor's – and the patient's – understanding of medical intervention. Precisely *when* the doctor intervened – whether he intervened at a particular hour or another, when to act and when to leave well alone – was in a sense the most important question. Such

---

[1] 'Hippocrates', *Aphorisms* 1.1, 68 Loeb (IV.458 L.).

decisions were taken to be potentially life-saving or fatal; and they were hotly debated, including, as we shall see, at the patient's bedside. The progress of a disease, too, can be analysed into different *kairoi* – significant or crucial moments in its development. This *kairos* or 'moment', then, according to the Hippocratic aphorism, is '*ōkus*'. The most obvious translation of this word is 'swift' or, as here, 'fleeting'; the adjective also has the connotations of 'acute' (in the particular context of disease) and 'sharp'. The relevance of that last possible translation – the sense in which the *kairos* was, indeed, for ancient doctors and patients, something *sharp* – will become clear in the ensuing paragraphs.

Krisis, which in ordinary Greek means 'judgement', 'assessment' or 'decision', acquired a technical medical sense, related to the course of an acute illness, usually a fever. Such illnesses were conceived as reaching their *krisis* at a certain moment, which was to say that that moment was *decisive*, it *determined* or *judged* the outcome of the illness, whether in a positive or a negative direction; it was the turning-point. And this *krisis* was in turn related to the 'intensification' (*paroxusmos*) of the fever, the moment at which, after a period of comparative normality, its symptoms became, briefly, highly intense, which was itself followed by a period of relaxation. This *paroxusmos* – in what follows translated 'episode' – in some cases brings on the *krisis*, which itself tends to be accompanied by a dramatic change, especially an evacuation of some sort.

It is worth noting, too, in this summary of the ancient and Galenic clinical approach to fevers, and their progress over given time periods, that the course of a disease can be analysed in terms of a four-part division: beginning, growth, peak, and post-peak. That division tells us something about the theoretical way in which a disease entity was conceptualized, as well as providing a rather striking point of contact with the analysis of times of life in chapter 2: in a way, the same kind of schematic analysis is applicable to both the growing (and declining) human organism and the pathological entity which afflicts it.[2]

Much more could be said about the long history and the rich semantic range of both terms, *kairos* and *krisis*, as they appear in a variety of literary, rhetorical, technical and legal contexts in ancient literature – and indeed about their relationship with each other. This is not the place for such a detailed survey,[3] but it will be instructive for our further investigation to highlight a few specific points.

---

[2] The four terms in Greek are *archē, auxēsis, akmē, parakmē* (the last two could also be translated 'prime' and 'post-prime' – as indeed has been my practice when they occur in the context of human ages, as in the texts discussed in the previous chapter): see *Crises* 1.2, 69,9–10 Alexanderson (IX.551 K.). I am grateful to Glen Cooper for drawing my attention to this parallel.
[3] For the history and range of senses of the term *kairos* from earliest times to late antiquity (with reference also to *krisis*) see Sipiora and Baumlin (2002); Trédé-Boulmer (2015); Longhi (2020).

First, *kairos* and its cognates are not only, or not even primarily, connected with time, in their earliest occurrences. Nor is the term by any means confined to medical or technical contexts. Rather, it has a very broad application, especially in rhetorical and philosophical literature, where its core semantic range involves the sense of appropriateness, of correct or fine judgement, of decisiveness. (The broader, not narrowly temporal, meaning is in play also in a number of texts of the Hippocratic corpus, where the sense is not always that of the correct *moment* for an intervention, but for example also of the correct amount or usage of certain foods or drugs.[4])

Secondly, there is in many contexts an important sense of briefness, of evanescence, of a moment to be seized appropriately or lost forever. Relevant here is the representation of *kairos* in ancient art. (See figure 11.) *Kairos* appears in a number of ancient statues – and, rather more clearly, descriptions of such statues – personified as a beautiful male youth, winged, with flowing locks, engaged in the use of pair of scales, holding a knife, and himself precariously balanced on the ground. Whatever the precise significance or connotations of these depictions, it seems clear that the personified *Kairos* combines the notions of the swiftness of the passing moment, of balance, of decisive action, and of precariousness – especially precariousness in the performance of an art.[5] Finally, that association with a knife may have a deeper significance. At least one plausible account of the term's etymology links it to a word for cutting; and indeed it seems likely that the word *krisis* should be connected with that same root.[6]

---

4 For this sense of *kairos* as corresponding to the correct measure or good proportion see Trédé-Boulmer (2015): 56–71. For such a sense in the Hippocratic corpus see e. g. *Regimen in Acute Diseases* 53–4, 108 Loeb (II.342 L.); *Affections* 53, 72 Loeb (VI.264 L.); *Diseases* 4.44, 132 Loeb (VII.566 L.) and 4.49, 144 Loeb (VII.578 L.).

5 For discussion and a full account of the ancient artistic representations see Trédé-Boulmer (2015): 75–81. The specific style of representation described here seems to go back to an original by Lysippus in the fourth century BCE, which obviously inspired both copies and literary responses; there are further depictions, with a less clearly defined activity or context, in a number of mosaics. A fifth-century hymn by Ion, as cited by Pausanias 5.14.9, is addressed to 'Kairos, most recent child of Zeus', and his possible inclusion amongst the gods is attested elsewhere, *Anthologia Palatina* 10.52.

In this context see also Csapo and Miller (1998), who suggest a social or political significance to *kairos*, arguing that it has connotations of newness and unpredictably, in some sense representing a democratic, unpredictable form of time in contradistinction to the established, unchanging, aristocratic norms of archaic Greek society.

6 See Trédé-Boulmer (2015): 51–3, linking καιρός to the root *kr–, from which are derived the verb κείρω, as well as a number of other words connected with the sense of cutting – and, indeed, the verb κρίνω and noun κρίσις with an original or early sense of 'separating', and therefore 'deciding'.

The notion of cutting is, perhaps, combined with the others already considered in the term's underlying – or at least in its early – understanding, and at the same time this is an understanding which connects it with the other term, *krisis*. To act in accordance with the *kairos* is to make crucial or decisive cut, at precisely the right time or place. A *kairos* is swift or 'sharp' in the sense that the relevant moment, like the sharpness of the knife, has a precision, a disappearing quality, which eludes the senses. And to act – or fail to act – in accordance with that *kairos* is something potentially decisive, something which will decide (*krinein*) a vital – or fatal – outcome. The two terms seem thus inextricably linked, not just in their later technical medical usage, but at a profound conceptual level from a much earlier time.

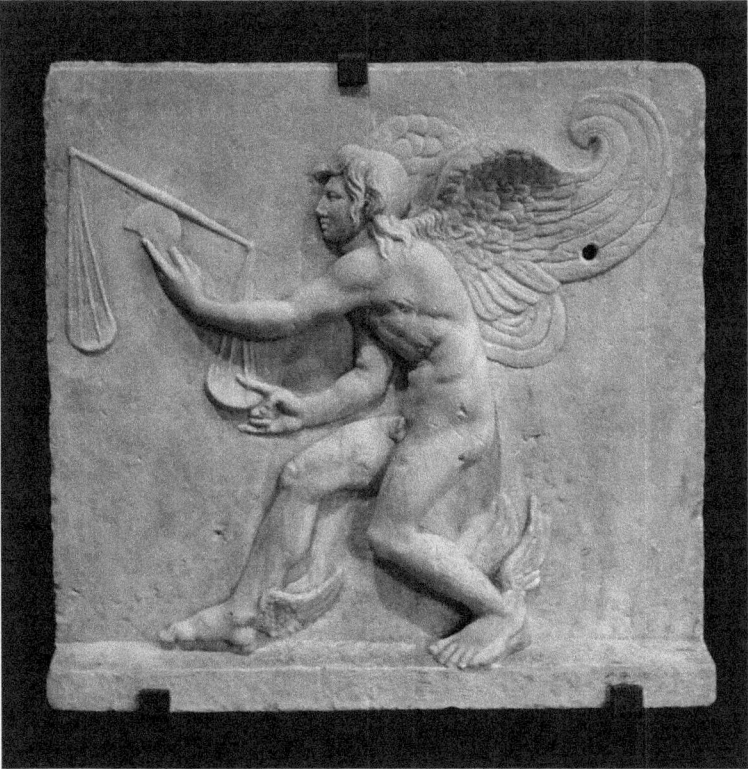

Figure 11: *Kairos* personified as a dashing youth, with a knife and scales, Roman copy of statue by Lysippus, Turin, Museum of Antiquities. Image source: http://ancientrome.ru/art/art worken/img.htm?id=2638

A little more – apart from the above connection with *kairos* – may be said about *krisis*, too. The term has a semantic range beyond (and informing) the technical medical one, where it encompasses the notions of assessment, of decision, especially a crucial or fateful decision, and of judgement, including judgement in a specifically legal sense. In the latter context, the noun and the related verb *krinein* may refer to a judicial sentence, in some cases a capital one. When, then, it is stated that a certain day *krinei* ('judges', 'decides', 'determines') a disease, these senses of fateful decision-making and judicial sentence form a crucial background to the ancient understanding of the term in that medical context.[7]

We see then the close connection, both in a broad Greek conceptual sense and in a technical medical context, between *kairos* and *krisis*, and the connection of both to the notions of speed, evanescence, urgency, correct and decisive judgement, skill, and peril.

We should note, finally, the connection of both to the third member or our Hippocratic trio cited above, *peira* – trial, testing, experience. Now that we have explored some of the connotations of the two other terms, we can see both how closely related to them is this notion of testing or experience – and also how relevant, in such a context, is that word applied to it in our initial aphoristic quotation: 'precarious'.[8]

Periodic diseases

The episodes of fevers were understood as taking place according to certain clearly defined periodic cycles or patterns (*periodoi, tupoi*). Such an understanding seems to have been fairly universal in Graeco-Roman medicine, although there were certainly – as we shall see later – disputes on the detail.

Moreover, it is difficult to overestimate the importance of fevers within ancient medical experience. They are a central feature of the Hippocratic texts,

---

[7] On both the medical sense and wider connotations of the term see Galen, *Commentary on Hippocrates' Prognostic* 3.6, 329 Heeg (XVIIIB.321–2 K.), who indeed highlights the connection of the medical to the juridical sense; the connection is made also at *Critical Days* 1.1 (IX.772 K.), where Galen likens the experience of the patient undergoing the *krisis* to that of one awaiting judgement on a capital charge. The technical medical sense of the critical day, the day on which a fever reaches its *krisis*, i.e. is 'decided', is already present in the Hippocratic corpus: see e.g. *Aphorisms* 2.23–4, 112–14 Loeb (IV.476 L.); *Prognostic* 20, 42 Loeb (II.168 L.).

[8] It is worth noting the mediaeval and early modern scientific use of the (cognate) term *periculum* (more usually translated 'danger') to refer to a 'trial' in the sense of 'experiment'.

in particular *Epidemics*, as we have already seen in passing; in Galen's work, a large part of his writing on specifically clinical matters is dedicated to fevers: they occupy most of the treatise *The Therapeutic Method to Glaucon* as well as much of the magnum opus *The Therapeutic Method*, and they are the main topic not just of *The Distinct Types of Fever* but also of *Crises*, *Critical Days* and *Against those who have written on Patterns, or Periods* (henceforward, *Periods*). Moreover, given the close conceptual connection between fever and aberrations of the pulse in Galen's medical system, one of the major significances of his very large, and clinically crucial, body of work on the pulse must also be understood in terms of its relationship to fever. To emphasize the practical value and importance of this discourse, the centrality of the above set of works – those on crises and critical days in particular – is highlighted by Galen himself, in his account of his own clinical successes in *Prognosis*, where they are mentioned as the crucial body of works to study in order to gain skill in diagnosis and prognosis.

Here we should understand the peculiar position of prognosis in the ancient medical context. The value of the ability to *prognose* outcomes – both in the sense of predicting them, and in the sense of telling the patient something which is already the case before s/he reveals it to you – is emphasized both by the author of the Hippocratic *Prognostic* and by Galen in his commentary on that work. Such ability is an essential tool for the doctor in gaining the patient's trust.

> I believe that it is best for the doctor to practise foreknowledge (*pronoia*); for by foreknowing (*proginōskein*) and foretelling in the presence of the patient those things which are currently the case, those which have happened and those which are going to happen, and by giving an account of those things which the invalid has left out, he will be more strongly believed to understand what is going on with the patient; and so people will gain the confidence to entrust themselves to the doctor.[9]

This text, in conjunction with Galen's commentary, brings into very clear focus both the highly public nature of the doctor–patient encounter and what is at stake in it. 'Prognosis' (of which the two words glossed in the above extract are cognates) is a crucial feature of ancient medicine above all because its successful accomplishment will convince the patient – and the prospective patient – of one's skill and authority; it will instil confidence in the patient, making him or her more likely to follow one's instructions, but it will also bring more patients in the future. Indeed, we have already observed this dynamic in the texts from Ga-

---

9 'Hippocrates', *Prognostic* 1.1, 6 Loeb (II.110 L.)

len's *Prognosis* cited in the second chapter. As Galen remarks in another text: 'nothing is so useful as to predict the beginnings of the forthcoming episodes'.[10]

Fevers and their recurrence: Hippocrates; Galen; Galen's rivals

The prominence of fevers in the Graeco-Roman medical discourse has been related, doubtless with justification, to the prevalence of malaria and a variety of related infectious diseases in the ancient Mediterranean.[11]

I do not enter into this area of retrospective diagnosis here. For our purposes, it is important to recognize that, whatever its origin in a disease entity that would have been identifiable in a modern pathology laboratory, the discourse of prediction and intervention that it gave rise to, with its complex range of categories and chronological divisions, requires completely different tools for its analysis.

The existence and individual peculiarities of different fevers, including their division into four main classes – continuous, quotidian, tertian and quartan – were already recognized in Hippocratic texts.[12] I here use the traditional, established Latinized names, which are based on a number of days and an inclusive system of counting. That is to say, a 'quotidian' (daily) fever has a recurrence or episode every day; a 'tertian' (three-day) fever has one every other day; a 'quartan' (four-day) every three days. This broad categorization survived for centuries, although with many divergences and refinements of the scheme. Galen takes over the fundamental four-part division (though he will acknowledge other classes too), while – as we noted briefly in chapter 2 – departing from the Hippocratic picture of *The Nature of the Human Being* by associating each of the main intermittent types (i.e., all the above, but not the 'continuous') with a different predominant bodily fluid – yellow bile, black bile or phlegm – rather than attributing fever in general to an excess of bile.

In social and medical-historical terms, what follows should be understood against the broader background of medical competitions, rivalries and conflicts

---

10 *Periods* 1 (VII.479–80 K.).
11 See most recently Miller (2020).
12 For periodic theories of disease in the Hippocratic texts, see Smith (1981); Langholf (1990): 78–127; Lloyd (1979): 154–68; Cooper (2011b): 127–8.

over authority, which we have already observed in the context of our discussion of Galen's engagement with *palaioi* and the *neōteroi* in chapter 3.[13]

A few points should be noted at the outset about the nature of our sources, and borne in mind as we proceed. The first is that, once again, our evidence comes overwhelmingly from Galen, and that this is true both of evidence for Galen's own views and practice and for those of his contemporaries or close predecessors. Secondly, and relatedly, that in the latter case the evidence for the views and practice is predominantly extremely hostile: Galen relays the views of his rival practitioners in order to destroy them. Thirdly, that Galen makes a number of claims about what distinguishes him from these rivals – claims which we have to attempt to see beyond, if we wish to construct a clear and less biased picture. These are: (a) that his rivals produce mystification and unnecessary complexity, while he does not; (b) that his theories and practice are authentically grounded in the Hippocratic; (c) that they are based on clinical experience and represent the best way of doing justice to that.

I shall not attempt to address each of these claims systematically, as it were to argue with Galen about them. I shall proceed rather by explicating both Galen's system and – on the basis of Galen's criticism, which provides the fullest evidence for them – those of his rivals, in an attempt to make each of them as clear as possible for the reader's consideration.

Non-Galenic views: over-simplification and over-complication

The texts of Galen – alongside other sources for the practice of medicine in the Roman imperial period – present us with an intensely competitive intellectual and clinical environment, in which highly theoretical debates, but also debates of immediate and urgent clinical significance, took place both in public arenas and at the bedsides of patients. As already remarked, neither the basic concept of the periodicity of acute illnesses, nor its vital importance, seems to have been disputed by any of these practitioners. But that still left huge scope for conflict and debate on the detail. Alongside Galen's own complex theorization, the rivals to his views can be divided into two basic groups, one which aimed consciously at a simplification of the theoretical framework, the other which – at least in Galen's caricature – complicated and obfuscated it to a bewildering degree. The for-

---

[13] Further on the socio-medical background and Galen's 'performance' within that context, see Barton (1994a); Nutton (2013), who emphasizes the actual ancient success and popularity of Methodism as a sect; Mattern (2008); Gill, Whitmarsh and Wilkins (2009).

mer group was the Methodists; the latter is less clearly identifiable, and known only from Galen's account of them.[14]

We already encountered the Methodists in the previous chapter. There we noted the apparently wide appeal of their system of medicine, based on a minimalist conceptual framework and a departure from the requirements of years of training, elite education and familiarity with ancient debates and ancient authorities. We noted too the extreme hostility that Galen has towards them, for precisely those reasons. In the context of fevers and periodicity, this minimalist system emerges in the universal applicability of the concept of the 'diatritus' – literally, the 'third day'[15]. On this view, every fever will have a recurrence on the third day from its first occurrence – that is, again remembering the inclusive counting system, every other day. During this period, until that third-day recurrence, the patient must fast. Moreover, the precise hour of the original occurrence must be taken into account: if the original onset of symptoms was, say, 'at the eighth hour', then fasting must continue until that 'suspected hour' has passed on the third day. In short, food must be withheld for 48 hours from the original onset of symptoms.

This one-size-fits-all clinical system of course flies in the face of the medical tradition, and tends to undermine any value in the differential diagnoses – and complex attendant schemes of interlocking fevers of different kinds – in which Galen claims expertise. We already looked at some passages, from *Prognosis*, in which the Methodists are attacked for their stubborn adherence to this simplistic scheme – and are, according to Galen, refuted by the outcome (see pp. 28–9 above). Let us consider a text which confronts Galen's analysis with the Methodists diatritus system even more explicitly. It is also a text which presents, perhaps more vividly than any other, the social reality of medical conflict in the Graeco-Roman world – the extraordinarily public, and conflictual, nature of the debate which could take place at the patient's bedside, and the risks that a doctor might take, in terms of both the life of the patient and his standing with the family, in order to win the day.

---

14 The evidence for both groups presented below will be from the texts of Galen; in the case of the Methodists, his picture of their theoretical account in this area can be complemented by other sources, in particular the texts of the first/second-century-CE Greek author Soranus and those of the much later Latin author, Caelius Aurelianus, whose work is closely based on that of Soranus.

15 The term, an adjective, has often been translated 'three-day period', with the noun *periodos* taken as understood; Leith (2008) has shown that the noun assumed is in fact 'day' – although this makes little difference to the fundamental medical conception.

The context is a bedside battle over the correct treatment of young man of 25 who is suffering from an acute fever – in Galen's analysis, a 'continuous' one, with its first and most acute onsets at the eleventh hour each day – precipitated by over-exertion and emotional excitation. The case history is a long one. Galen introduces it as an account of 'a patient in whose case I first dared, led by reason, to put aside the "third day" [doctrine]', adding that his confidence grew on the basis of his success: 'when the first trial (*peira*) bears witness to [the truth of] the discoveries arrived at indicatively, it renders one more confident on the second occasion'.[16] By the time Galen arrives, on the third day, the patient has been subjected to the diatritus-led fasting regime and is in a perilous state; Galen gives food immediately, and continues to do so at various points on the following days. We take up the story on the eighth day, with Galen and his Methodist rivals still arguing, both over which of them has kept him alive thus far and over the appropriate interventions from now on. The passage is a remarkable one, giving a vivid real-life exemplification of those crucial conceptions with which we started, *kairos*, *krisis* and *peira*, and throwing into sharp relief the immediacy and urgency, as well as the highly public nature, of the clinical disputes between doctors – and the extraordinary nature of the risks undergone in the attempt to win them. (See figure 12.)

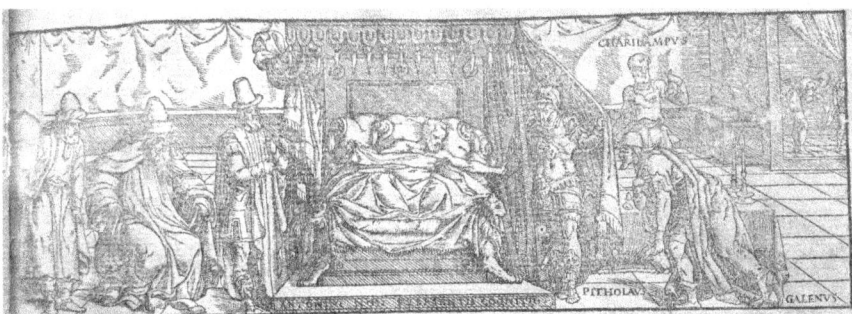

Figure 12: The bedside as battlefield: Galen correctly diagnosing the illness of the emperor Marcus Aurelius, surrounded by rival physicians. The image is based on Galen's own description of the event in *Prognosis*, and is from the frontispiece of A. Gadaldini's 1565 Juntine edition, *Galeni Opera Omnia quae extant, secundae classis libri*, Venice. My thanks to Lucia Raggetti for providing the reproduction

> At this point indeed their senselessness, or competitiveness, or whatever one wishes to call it, in instructing him to go beyond the third day in the first place, could be quite clearly

---

16 *The Therapeutic Method* 10.3 (X.671 K.).

understood. For it was absolutely plain to all that the man would not have survived until the fourth day if he had not been given nourishment before the episode on the third day; yet they still claimed that it was wrong to have fed him then, and on the successive days. But, of course, it was not possible to abandon the patient and not give food at the hour of the episode on each day, simply in order to refute these people.

I gave him nourishment in a similar way on the ninth day, and observed that during the episode the pulse was stronger than before, although it was still weak, and the extremities cool. I was now no longer able to endure the wretched babbling of the doctors, but on the eleventh day said in advance to the friends of the patient that they would understand today that he had thus far been saved by me, and instructed him to go beyond the time of the episode [without eating]. At this hour, then, there was a complete absence of a pulse and a severe cooling of the whole body, to the point where the patient could no longer speak, and was hardly conscious of being touched. I and all the doctors who had seen him from the beginning were called together, and we were in danger of being practically torn limb from limb by the family of the patient – I for deliberately abandoning his safety through the desire to win a contest, the lovers of the *diatritus* because of their ignorance and lack of perception. These latter in fact became paler and colder than the patient himself, and tried to devise a way of escape. But I had foreseen that, and ordered the outer door to be locked, instructing one of my followers to take the key and look after it.

I then came forward and said: 'Now, I suppose, you have already become convinced who it is who has saved this man so far; and he will again be saved by me. For I would not have refrained from feeding him during this episode if I had expected him to perish completely; rather, I realized that he had sufficient strength from the previous nourishment to be able to withstand the episode … But in order to refute these people, and to persuade some of you who have been listening to their claims … I shall, even though I have missed the correct moment (*kairos*), demonstrate to them that it is appropriate to nourish certain illnesses … So saying, I prised open his jaws and poured in three measures of thin gruel, using a narrow-mouthed vessel … At which point he opened his eyes and began to hear, speak and recognize those around him …'[17]

So, the Methodists obscure the truth – and risk disastrous clinical outcomes – through their excessive simplification, their rejection of the appropriate theoretical framework and distinctions.

On the other side, Galen mercilessly attacks others whose observations and calculations appear to have led them to excessive theoretical complexity.

Galen's own conceptual schemes (as well as his criticisms of others') are laid out most fully in *The Distinct Types of Fever*, in *Critical Days* and in *Periods*, and have been the subject of important recent analyses by Glen Cooper and Kassandra Miller.[18] As in so many other fields, Galen criticizes the proponents of rival schemes for both obfuscation and complication – in particular, here, for the in-

---

17 *The Therapeutic Method* 10.3 (X.675–7 K.)
18 See Cooper (2011a), (2013); Miller (2018), (2020).

troduction of categories beyond the three basic types of intermittent fevers well established in the tradition – and for failure to make distinctions in the correct manner.

> Not only have most doctors erred in the classes (*genē*) of distinctions, either producing an excessive number of them, so that they make mention of useless ones, or an insufficient number, passing over some of the useful ones; they have, equally, blundered in the division (*tomē*) within the classes, into proper distinct types (*diaphorai*).[19]

It is worth noting, in relation to our discussion in the last chapter, that such criticism is again couched in terms of the departure of such doctors from the clear picture given by Hippocrates (at this point Galen mentions the summary given in *Epidemics*, book 6).

In *Periods*, which again begins with an attack on the *neōteroi* for departing from tradition and from 'the accepted usage of the Greeks',[20] Galen elaborates in detail on one such kind of over-complication and mystification. Claiming both the medical tradition and the consensus of medically literate laypersons on his side, Galen acknowledges that an observed daily recurrence of a fever might correctly be interpreted as indicating the presence of a quotidian fever, or in some cases as the simultaneous presence of two tertians or of three quartans. We shall return to those Galenically admissible complexities later. For the moment, let us consider further the views that he is here attacking.

Presenting his own as the voice of common sense – as advocating a view that will be shared by the reasonably well-informed layperson – Galen suggests that a slightly earlier or later occurrence, in terms of the exact hour, need not be clinically significant: we can all learn to recognize a fever as 'quotidian', even if it does not recur at precisely the same hour each day. By contrast,

> those who are slaves to the hypotheses mentioned, when they encounter someone with an episode two hours earlier each day, state that the period is one of twenty-two hours, and the whole pattern not a simple one but some composite; then, after much enquiry and calculation amongst themselves, which they carry out either using their fingers or by reference

---

19 *The Distinct Types of Fever* 1.1 (VII.274 K.).
20 The immediate criticism here is on a linguistic point: not only have the moderns introduced the new term *tupos* ('pattern') in the context of periodic illness, they also insist on a terminological distinction, whereby the *tupos* is a sub-category of the *periodos* ('period'), namely that which consists in a number of *complete* days and nights, *Periods* 1 (VII.476 K.). Galen's argument in this text, and his complex calculations, summarized briefly below, are analysed in detail by Miller (2020).

to a table written in some book, they state that such a pattern is a '12-times dodecan'. When people who hear this laugh at them, they get angry.[21]

In Galen's explication of the rival view, he goes so far as to explain the mathematical procedure involved in their calculations in detail, with a number of examples, and to transcribe a conversion table to assist in such calculations. (See figure 13.) The practitioners in question identify a precise number of hours (H) as the period of the fever under examination. In the table, each main fever type (i.e., those defined in terms of a number of days, quotidian, tertian, etc.) is matched with the precise total number of hours (R) corresponding to that type. For example for the four-day or quartan fever type (since days are counted inclusively) the value of R is 72.[22] Galen devotes many words to detailed explication of the calculation, but it seems that it may essentially be summarized as follows. We take the precise number of hours (H) of the period. We calculate what fraction H is of a main fever type, i.e. one defined in terms of a number of days. This is done by finding in the table the first value of R of which H is a factor, and dividing R by H. The resulting figure is combined with the day-type to give the correct formula for the more precise fever type. So, for example, if H is 8, this is 1/3 of 24, which is the value of R corresponding to the quotidian fever type; thus an observed period of 8 hours implies the presence of a '3-times quotidian' (i.e., one which will recur three times within the day). Or, in the example above, H is 22, which is 1/12 of 264, the value of R corresponding to the dodecan fever type (again, always remembering that we count inclusively).

---

21 Galen, *Periods* 1 (VII.477 K.). More precisely the Greek here speaks not of 'a 12-times dodecan', but of '12 dodecans', in the plural. I have thus departed slightly from the precise terminology that is attributed to these practitioners in the text, which, it seems to me, at least if understood literally, cannot correspond to the conceptual scheme being proposed. This is surely that there is *one* fever, which recurs at a period which is a fraction of the larger entity, the dodecan – i.e., it recurs at regular intervals *within* the overall 12-day cycle – rather than there is a plurality of 'dodecans', as Galen's text, taken literally, suggests. It seems possible that either (a) Galen has misrepresented their language or (b) distortion has found its way into the manuscript tradition, as a function of the rather unfamiliar mathematical conception it puts forward. Perhaps, rather than 'twelve dodecans' (etc.) we should read 'a twelfth of a dodecan' (etc.). While reserving judgement on this question, and not necessarily suggesting that emendation is required, I have opted for this compromise translation, which at least gives the required sense of a single fever recurring repeatedly within a larger cycle, as well as perhaps also getting across some of the perceived oddity of the notion. I am grateful to Kassandra Miller for discussion of this passage and this problem by e-mail.
22 See *Periods* 4–7, VII.488–512 K., with the conversion table at VII.490–3 K.

So, we have a '12-times dodecan' (one which will recur 12 times within the longer 12-day period).

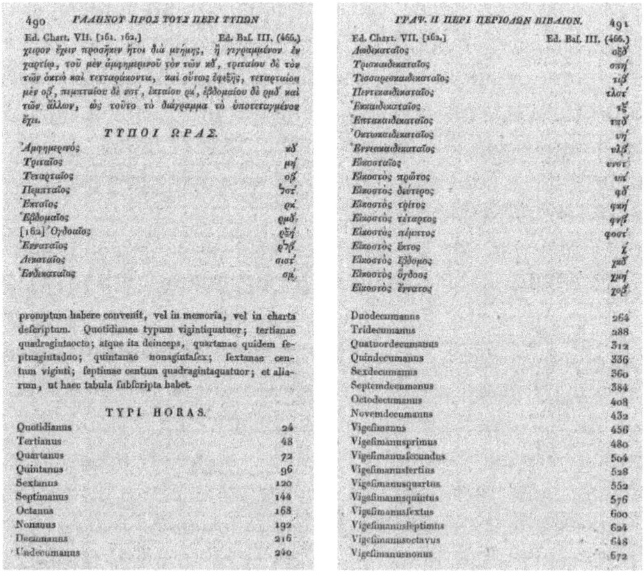
490 ΓΑΛΗΝΟΥ ΠΡΟΣ ΤΟΥΣ ΠΕΡΙ ΤΥΠΩΝ

Ed. Chart. VII. [161. 162.] Ed. Bas. III. (466.)

χειρον ἔχειν προσῆκεν ἤτοι διὰ μνήμης, ἢ γεγραμμένον ἐν χαρτίῳ, τοῦ μὲν ἀμφημερινοῦ τὸν τῶν κδ΄, τριταίου δὲ τὸν τῶν ὀκτὼ καὶ τετταράκοντα, καὶ οὕτως ἐφεξῆς, τεταρταίου μὲν οβ΄, πεμπταίου δὲ ϟϛ΄, ἑκταίου ρκ΄, ἑβδομαίου δὲ ρμδ΄ καὶ τῶν ἄλλων, ὡς τοῦτο τὸ διάγραμμα τὸ ὑποτεταγμένον ἔχει.

ΤΥΠΟΙ	ΩΡΑΣ.
Ἀμφημερινός	κδ΄
Τριταῖος	μη΄
Τεταρταῖος	οβ΄
Πεμπταῖος	ϟϛ΄
Ἑκταῖος	ρκ΄
Ἑβδομαῖος	ρμδ΄
[162] Ὀγδοαῖος	ρξη΄
Ἐνναταῖος	ρϟβ΄
Δεκαταῖος	σιϛ΄
Ἑνδεκαταῖος	σμ΄

promptum habere convenit, vel in memoria, vel in charta descriptum. Quotidianae typum vigintiquatuor; tertianae quadragintaocto; atque ita deinceps, quartanae quidem septuagintaduo; quintanae nonagintasex; sextanae centum viginti; septimae centum quadragintaquatuor; et aliarum, ut haec tabula subscripta habet.

TYPI	HORAS.
Quotidianus	24
Tertianus	48
Quartanus	72
Quintanus	96
Sextanus	120
Septimanus	144
Octanus	168
Nonanus	192
Decimanus	216
Undecumanus	240

ΓΡΑΨ. Η ΠΕΡΙ ΠΕΡΙΟΔΩΝ ΒΙΒΛΙΟΝ. 491

Ed. Chart. VII. [162.] Ed. Bas. III. (466.)

Δωδεκαταῖος	σξδ΄
Τρισκαιδεκαταῖος	σπη΄
Τεσσαρεσκαιδεκαταῖος	τιβ΄
Πεντεκαιδεκαταῖος	τλϛ΄
Ἑκκαιδεκαταῖος	τξ΄
Ἑπτακαιδεκαταῖος	τπδ΄
Ὀκτωκαιδεκαταῖος	υη΄
Ἐννεακαιδεκαταῖος	υλβ΄
Εἰκοσταῖος	υνϛ΄
Εἰκοστὸς πρῶτος	υπ΄
Εἰκοστὸς δεύτερος	φδ΄
Εἰκοστὸς τρίτος	φκη΄
Εἰκοστὸς τέταρτος	φνβ΄
Εἰκοστὸς πέμπτος	φοϛ΄
Εἰκοστὸς ἕκτος	χ΄
Εἰκοστὸς ἕβδομος	χκδ΄
Εἰκοστὸς ὄγδοος	χμη΄
Εἰκοστὸς ἔννατος	χοβ΄

Duodecumanus	264
Tridecumanus	288
Quatuordecumanus	312
Quindecumanus	336
Sexdecumanus	360
Septemdecumanus	384
Octodecumanus	408
Novemdecumanus	432
Vigesimanus	456
Vigesimanusprimus	480
Vigesimanussecundus	504
Vigesimanustertius	528
Vigesimanusquartus	552
Vigesimanusquintus	576
Vigesimanussextus	600
Vigesimanusseptimus	624
Vigesimanusoctavus	648
Vigesimanusnonus	672

Figure 13: Calculating the period (wrongly): part of the conversion table in Galen's *Periods*, from Kühn's edition (vol. VII). The left-hand column on each page contains fever types, defined as numbered days from the inception of the illness (e. g. 3rd = tertian ('tertianus'), 4th = quartan ('quartanus'), 12th = dodecan ('duodecumanus'), etc.), the right-hand column the total number of hours corresponding to each of these types. (Original Greek text above, Latin translation below.) Galen's rival practitioners proceed by identifying the precise number of hours (H) of the disease's 'period', then locating the first number in the right-hand column (R) of which H is a factor, then dividing R by H. The resulting figure is combined with the corresponding fever type in the left-hand column to produce the precise fever type, e. g. if H = 22, the formula is '12-times' dodecan because 22 is 264/12 (and is not a factor of any previous value in column R).

Here, as Miller observes, Galen takes the opportunity not only to show off his mathematical facility, but to attack the system on the basis of a fundamental apparent flaw, namely that such calculations can be carried out in more than one way. For example, if the period is one of 12 hours, the result yielded could be a '2-times quotidian', a '4-times tertian', a '6-times quartan', and so on. Galen follows the thought process and conceptual scheme in detail, apparently enabling the reader too to produce diagnoses and prognoses in accordance with it, before rejecting it as valueless.

Galen's own schemes

As already suggested, Galen is keen in the above context to present his own voice as one of common sense, speaking against the obfuscations of his contemporaries, which are criticized on two main grounds: (a) the fact that they pay excessive attention to unimportant detail, in this case the precise hour of the onset, when this differs somewhat on successive days; (b) the fact that their conceptual system leads to more than one possible answer on the basis of the same data.

It is interesting to bear these criticisms in mind while moving to a consideration of Galen's own conceptual scheme.

The basic categories have already been outlined: those of the continuous fever, the quotidian, the tertian and the quartan. There are, however, further subdivisions and attendant complexities. First, fevers may be 'static' or 'moving' – that is, they may, in the latter case, vary in the moment of their recurrence within a given day. So, Galen himself uses as a diagnostic criterion the very feature which he criticizes the *neōteroi* for paying excessive attention to in the elaboration of *their* diagnostic scheme. Secondly – and as we already observed in passing in the first chapter – one may have two, or even more, fevers (including fevers of more than one type) concurrently. By allowing these two sets of possibilities – so that we may have the simultaneous action of two or more fevers, of different periodicities and different times of first onset, *and* those periodicities do not have to consist of a precise 24-hour time-span – Galen is surely also allowing (though by no means openly admitting) a wealth of possible interpretive solutions to his own recorded sets of data.

The complexity and fluidity of Galen's system is brilliantly displayed in a passage in *Crises*, where we find not only that there is a simultaneous occurrence of three tertians, but also that they are irregular or 'moving' tertians; Miller gives a table setting out the precise data which Galen claims here to have observed, emphasizing their close connection with precise hourly time-keeping, and setting them in relationship with his theoretical interpretation of them.[23] It seems undeniable, though, that the criticism levelled by Galen at the *neōteroi*, for their calculation of such absurd collections of entities as a '12-times dodecan' – and above all for elaborating a system which admits of a plurality of interpretations of a given set of data – could very plausibly be turned back upon him by his opponents. One is tempted, indeed, to suggest that the possible variables in Galen's system make it much *more* complex than those he criticizes, and also –

---

23 *Crises* 2.9, 151–3 Alexanderson (IX.680–3 K.); Miller (2020): 276–9.

crucially – allow him to be the ultimate arbiter between different possible interpretations of the apparently messy and polysemic data.

Such polysemicity, and the related arrogation to himself of the expertise required to make the correct judgement on the basis of the data and the conceptual system, are arguably a central feature of what is going on in the Galenic text. It is difficult here not to be drawn to Barton's analysis of ancient medical and astrological texts in terms of the multiplicity of interpretations allowed by the conceptual framework validated by the practitioner, and of the flexibility and ultimate control that the practitioner thus reserves to himself.[24]

A final observation may be made in this context, namely that Galen's analytical schemes themselves admit of some fluidity and variation, at least in their manner of exposition. In spite of the strong insistence on the correct identification of the critical day in the texts discussed above, Galen makes no explicit mention of that concept in another central work on the analysis of periodic disease, *Crises*. Here, by contrast, the focus is on the four-phase analysis – beginning, growth, peak, post-peak – mentioned above (p. 103 with n. 2).

Whatever view one takes, however, of the consistency of Galen's conceptual schemes, or of the relative strengths of them and those of his unnamed rivals – or whether one feels the need to take a view on these matters at all – the schemes themselves give ample evidence of the importance of time measurement, of calculations based on it, and of their contested nature, in ancient medical culture.

Reconciling theory, observation and authority: Galen's medical month

Another ramification of this intricate calculation and use of time units in Graeco-Roman medicine is Galen's invention and employment of the 'medical month' – an invention which represents at once perhaps his most original and individualistic contribution in this area, and also the most bizarre development, causing perplexity to scholars of the early modern period as it may still to us today.[25]

---

24 Cf. the analysis of Barton (1994a), in the context not only of medicine but also of physiognomics and astrology.
25 For a more detailed account of Galen's theory and calculation here see Cooper (2011a), (2011b), the latter in particular highlighting the superficial and apparently ill-thought-through employment by Galen of astrological theory and explanations; Heilen (2018); for the subsequent reception of his account see the latter and Cooper (2013).

Galen is led down this pathway by a particular problem – one which arises in part, again, from that commitment to the Hippocratic texts which we have already seen to be central to his medical thinking. The problem is not one of reconciling Hippocratic authority with observed experience: these, in Galen's view, are perfectly in harmony. It is rather that of reconciling *both* those with the mathematical implications of the scheme of periodic recurrence of tertians and quartans, already outlined.

The difficultly, simply stated, is this. In the progress of a tertian fever, Hippocrates emphasizes the importance of the 20th day: it is, in fact, one of the most important 'critical days'. And this is borne out, according to Galen, by observed fact. Yet, on a calculation based on the recurrence of a fever every other day, it is not the 20th but the 21st day which should be relevant. What is it that can explain the discrepancy?

Here, Galen enters into an intricate – and one is tempted to think, improvised – mathematical argument, based partly on established astronomical and astrological measurements and explanations, and partly on his own ratiocination. The passage in question, from book 3, chapter 9 of Galen's *Critical Days*, in fact represents the only serious discussion of astrology in his work, and the discussion, as has been argued in recent scholarship, appears rather extraneous to his usual modes of explanation. Nevertheless, both the fact that he does engage seriously with astrology, and the particular use to which he puts it – one which was to be of considerable influence, as well as source of considerable debate, in later centuries – are of considerable interest.

Galen presents the motions of the heavenly bodies, or their precise positions during the month, as providing the underlying explanation for the periodicity of fevers. *Why* should a fever be more virulent at one time of the month and less so at others, and what explains the regularity? The solution is to be sought in the effects of the moon and of other heavenly bodies, and the chronological pattern of these effects therefore discovered through a precise calculation and subdivision of the month, understood in terms of the progress of the moon through the zodiac. Different zodiacal signs, in conjunction with the moon, have different effects on the human body; the precise point of the latter in the monthly cycle will have important physical, and sometimes pathological, effects.[26]

So, what Galen is here presenting is not a justification of astrology in general terms, but a rationalizing astrology, whereby it is thought plausible that the plan-

---

26 For the fundamental understanding of the heavenly motions which forms the background to these astrological notions see above, pp. 52–4 with figure 7. For detail on how the positions of the heavenly bodies in relation to the zodiac are defined and analysed in ancient astrological theory see Barton (1994b), ch. 4.

ets and constellations have distinct physical effects on us at different times of the month, as a function of their physical characteristics and our own bodily dispositions. This broad methodological approach, whereby actions of the heavenly bodies on human lives are explained in physical terms, and considered as part of the same causal scheme that also includes geographical, meteorological and anthropological phenomena, is sometimes known as 'natural astrology'. A parallel may be drawn here with Ptolemy, whose employment of astrological theory is, however, of course, highly sophisticated in comparison with Galen's. It is worth noting in this context that Galen equates the traditional terms 'beneficent' or 'maleficent', as applied to planets, with the categories 'well-mixed' (*eukratos*) and 'badly-mixed' (*duskratos*). While expounding (a very simplified version of) traditional astrological theory, he is simultaneously at pains to draw the heavenly bodies in question into his standard model of explanation, that based on the fundamental physical qualities and their mixture.[27]

Seeking such an explanation, then, on the one hand, and on the other exercised to find a justification for the fact that the 20th, and not the 21st, day tends to be critical, Galen arrives at the following solution. First of all, in considering the course of the moon through the sky, and the relationship between this and the human subject, there are two possible 'month' units that could be thought relevant: the sidereal month, that is the time it takes for the moon to return to a similar position in relation to the fixed stars, and the synodic month, that is the time it takes to return to the same observed position in relation to the earth. The former is a period of 27 1/3 days, the latter one of 29 1/2 days.

It is at this point that Galen injects his original contribution. In order to arrive at the relevant 'medical month', he first subtracts three days from the synodic month, thus arriving at a figure of 26 1/2 days, and then takes the mean of this and the sidereal month. The resultant figure is one of 26 11/12 days.

Galen has two intellectual motivations here. He is attempting to give an account which is plausible in physical terms, an account, that is, which does justice to what he takes to be the active physical powers of the moon upon earthly subjects. Though the physical theory here is far from clearly explained or elaborated, he does make *some* attempt at such an explanation, in terms of the 'alteration of the air around the earth' performed by the heavenly bodies in the monthly cycle.[28] At the same time, the Hippocratic texts and his own observa-

---

[27] '... the moon naturally indicates what the days will be like, not just to sick people but to the healthy. If it stands in conjunction with the well-mixed (*eukratous*) planets, which are also called beneficent, it makes them good; if with the badly-mixed (*duskratous*), bad' (*Critical Days* 3.6, IX.911–12 K.).
[28] *Critical Days* 3.9 (IX.930 K.)

tions lead him to believe that a correct calculation of the lunar cycle must somehow yield the result that a critical moment comes on the 20th day. This solution meets both needs. The justification of the diminution of the synodic month is that the number of days subtracted corresponds to the period in which the moon is invisible from earth through its conjunction with the sun (i. e., the period of the new moon), during which it cannot be thought to exert any physical powers upon us.

If we proceed, then, from this medical month of 26 11/12 days, we arrive at a proportionally shortened week, too; and it is this shortened week, again, which should be taken as relevant to the periodicity of fevers. The end of the first such week will take us to a point 6 days, 17 1/2 hours from the start of the month; the end of the second, to 13 days, 11 hours; the third, to 20 days, 4 1/2 hours; the fourth, to 26 days, 22 hours.[29]

The end of the third such week, then, or to put it another way the completion of the seventh three-day period, will take us to a point 20 days and a few hours from the relevant start point; in most cases, then, though this will depend upon the exact hour of the first occurrence of the fever, the episode will recur on the 20th, not the 21st, day.

Another way of looking at it, then, is that the length of the *day* must be recalculated at slightly more than 23 hours, and that it is to this 23-and-a-bit-hour day that we must look as the relevant unit against which to observe the recurrence. We are again in a realm in which the precise hour of recurrence of fever on a day should, in principle at least, be carefully observed, and where an intricate calculation is required for the assessment of its true significance – again, rather to the contrary of Galen's relaxed marks about slippage by a couple of hours in the recurrence of fevers, observed above. It seems, however, that such implications of the system are not by any means implemented in full, or borne in mind by Galen in his discussions of fevers in general.

Incidentally, the question *how* patient or doctor is to pay such close attention to the precise number of the hours – the question, that is, which we raised in the first chapter, and to which we will return in the next, of the extent to which actual measuring devices were used and relied upon – is not explicitly raised, let alone answered, by our texts. We may probably take it that complete accuracy of time measurement, at least measurement more precise than that afforded by a reasonably recent inspection of a sundial, was not considered particularly impor-

---

29 These complicated fractions, made more complicated by the laborious ancient Greek way of describing them, unsurprisingly became somewhat garbled at points in the manuscript tradition; the situation is described in detail by Heilen (2018), who also offers a restored version of the most relevant part of the text of IX.932 Kühn.

tant, in relation to a scheme which, after all, is not attempting to subdivide the hours. (We shall observe in the final chapter one particular medical context in which much smaller units apparently *were* apparently measured.) It remains a possibility, however, especially in the elite households which are, after all, the milieu in which an educated doctor like Galen practised, that sophisticated water clocks were indeed consulted for the purpose of ensuring that the 'suspected hour' had definitely passed.

In any case, the process of conversion necessitated by this system – the conversion of actual days into 'medical' days – was attempted in early modern times, and conversion tables produced,[30] although it seems unclear how widespread the attempt to employ Galen's complex astrologically-based model was in practice.

Certainly, Galen's *Critical Days*, the passage discussed above in particular, were much discussed in mediaeval and early modern times. The debate over astrological medicine raged, with this text a central bone of contention. Some argued for the fundamentals of Galen's position, while suggesting that his understanding of astrology needed to be improved, with a rejection of Galen in this context in favour of Ptolemy; others, that astrology had no place in medicine; still others wanted to defend Galen's position wholesale.[31]

Indeed, it is difficult to imagine that Galen's apparently improvised theory did not attract criticism from the first moment at which he stated it; and it would be fascinating to have his response to such criticism. The particular text in question, and the theoretical problems raised, require further scholarly analysis.[32] But it is very difficult to see how the inactivity of the moon for three days at the end of the month's cycle could be thought to provide a model with any sort of general applicability. If the medical month concludes, as Galen wishes, in 26.9 days, then this presumably means that the monthly cycle starts again from that same point. Obvious objections to this are, first, that it does not in fact start then, because the moon has not, in *any* astronomical

---

[30] For example by a Bolognese professor of mathematics, Antonio Magni, whose conversion table is discussed and reproduced by Heilen (2018): 233–5.

[31] A number of positions in the early modern response are laid out in detail by Cooper (2013), considering the reactions of such figures as Girolamo Cardano, Pietro d'Abano, Girolamo Fracastoro, Pico della Mirandola, Giovanni Mainardi, Nicolas Oresme and Thomas Bodier. See also Pennuto (2008).

[32] But see the literature cited in notes 25 and 31 above. Further aspects of Galen's analysis here are his distinction between 'general' and 'specific' influences of the moon, and the relationship between solar and lunar influence; but it remains unclear how these elements are incorporated in a coherent causal account. I am grateful to Glen Cooper for further discussions and personal communications on this undoubtedly puzzling topic.

sense, returned to its original position at that point; secondly, that the moon must – *ex hypothesi* – be from a medical point of view inactive for the next three days, and therefore *not* starting a new cycle. What, then, happens to the cycle, from a clinical point of view, from that point on? It would seem to need a 'reset', where everything stops for three days and then cyclical influence begins again – but what possible clinical sense could that make, for someone actually experiencing a fever?

Galen might, perhaps, feel able to ignore that objection, on the grounds that in practice all fevers terminate their activity, or their periodicity, within a single month. But there seems to be a third, even more fundamental, objection, namely that the model seems in the first place only designed for cases where the first onset of the fever coincides with the beginning of the moon's cycle; otherwise that inactive period will fall somewhere in the middle of the month, and this seems to make nonsense of the whole model. It is, perhaps, not even clear what it would mean for the moon to cease its activity in the middle of the periodic fever that it is supposedly in some sense causally determining; but presumably this would at the very least upset the usual periodic calculation.

Whether or not Galen had a ready response to such objections, however, his attempt to create new time units to assist in the explanation of observed cyclical patterns constitutes yet another striking example of the significance and complexity of time measurement in relation to medical diagnosis and clinical practice in the ancient world. And one which cast a long shadow.

Chapter Five:
Time, motion, rhythm: reality, perception and quantification

In this chapter I look at discussions of the fundamental nature, both of time itself and of its perception and measurability. Here again medical writing, that of Galen especially, draws upon existing philosophical debates. It introduces perspectives which enrich those debates themselves, while also shedding light on ancient approaches to the challenges of the measurement of time in relation to motion – of the assessment of speed, frequency and rhythm. The value of a study of Galen's – and other medical, as well as musical – discussions, then, is not just that they engage with and contribute in interesting and unexpected ways to the philosophical debate. Such discussions also make clear the relevance of the abstract conceptions in real-life contexts – for example in clinical contexts, as well as in relation to the practical challenges of the assessment of time, speed or rhythm. We shall begin with the more abstract, theoretical analyses, before moving to a consideration of some of these practical significances, in both musical and medical contexts.

Most of Galen's discussions in this area, indeed, consider related questions conjointly – the nature of time, the relationship of time to space and motion, the nature of our perception of these – and arise in the context of enquiries related to clinical practice, specifically that concerning the accurate discernment or measurement of the motions of the pulse. There is also a series of remarks of a more theoretical nature, which are available to us in the form of 'fragments' – that is to say, as statements attributed to Galen, either as verbatim quotations or in indirect form, by later authors, unfortunately shorn of their original argumentative context. We shall proceed by considering first this more theoretical – and harder to interpret – material before moving to the discussions in the treatises on the pulse, which we shall consider alongside evidence for the related theories of the earlier pulse theorist Herophilus of Chalcedon. There, we shall be considering the principles and processes involved in the measurement of very small time units, and also of ratios between time units, as reflected in ancient medical evidence of attempts to measure speed or rhythm. Throughout, the question arises of the relative or absolute basis of the measurements, and of the extent – or limits – of any attempts at quantification.

First, let us give a very brief account of the relevant previous tradition of theoretical discussions of time.

Philosophical questions and the relationship of time to motion

The Greek philosophical tradition centres on a number of core problems or paradoxes regarding time. Is time real? Is it continuous or atomic in its structure? Is time a kind of motion, and if not what is the relationship between the two? How is time related to eternity? Is the existence of time in some sense dependent on the human observer? How can we understand or define a moment of time, or the relationship of the present to the past and future?[1]

I offer here a highly simplified account of, as it were, the key moments in the history of this philosophical discourse.

Plato made a fundamental distinction between eternity (*aiōn*) and time (*chronos*), related to his distinction of the ideal or intellectual realm from the mutable, physical one of everyday observation and experience. Eternity involves no change; time is a feature of the world of coming-to-be (*genesis*) rather than that of true being, that is of the physical, perceptible world: it arises as a function of the creation of the cosmos, the heavenly bodies and their motions coming about as the instruments of its measurement. Relatedly, the perception or measurement of time, and perhaps even time itself, only exist in relation to a human observer.[2]

This latter thought is taken further in the subsequent Platonic tradition, especially by Plotinus, for whom eternity and time can be seen as corresponding to two modes of existence, the former that of the Intellect, to which human beings strive to return, the latter played out in our ordinary, materially conditioned, lives.[3] Time, for Plotinus, is 'the life of the soul in a movement that changes from one way of life to another' (*Enneads* 3.7.11.43–5). Central here is the notion of time as dependent on, or a feature of, human life – more specifically, of the

---

[1] Still fundamental here is Sorabji (1983), following these and other philosophical topics concerned with time from classical Greek to mediaeval times.
[2] In the *Timaeus*, time is created as an image of eternity, as a concomitant of the creation of the universe; the division into time units – and indeed that into past, present and future – are a function of the human observer and of physical motion and change (37d–38b). (Cf. the characterization of time as 'an image of eternity moving according to number', κατ' ἀριθμὸν ἰοῦσαν αἰώνιον εἰκόνα, *Timaeus* 37d6–7.) The sun, moon and planets come into being for the demarcation and monitoring of time (38c–39e). As we shall see, this gives rise to an interpretive question: is time in some sense a feature or function of physical motion – dependent upon it for its existence – or is rather simply that by which motion is measured?
[3] Plotinus elaborates his views on time and eternity (also giving a substantial account of the previous tradition) in his *Ennead* 3.7; for further analysis see Beierwaltes (1967), Smith (1996), Tempest-Walters (2020).

restless human soul feeling the need to depart from unity and eternity – rather than as something existing independently of us. Nevertheless, Plotinus is clear that time is not itself a motion but 'that within which physical motion takes place'. Here he is rejecting a view – and an interpretation of Plato – apparently widespread amongst Platonic commentators, according to which time is, indeed, a kind of motion – the motion of the 'whole', or of the 'sphere'.[4] Aristotle too, as we shall see shortly, suggests that the view of time as a form of motion is that most widespread in his milieu.

The motivation for such a view is apparently that the revolutions of the heavenly bodies, or of the whole sphere, provide a constant against which time is measured. (For the fundamental 'two-sphere' view underlying ancient astronomical observations and theories see above, pp. 52–4 and figure 7.) Plotinus objects to this, pointing to the different speeds of motion of different heavenly bodies, and arguing that therefore time measurement requires a standard external to *all* such bodies. Time does not, then, consist in their motion; rather, those bodies have been generated in order to make time manifest and delimited, in order for there to be a visible measure (*Enneads* 3.7.8; 3.7.12). Plotinus also argues that time is that by which we quantify rather than being itself quantifiable (here taking issue with Aristotle: *Physics* 4.11, 219b7–8 and 4.12, 220b8).

Of course there is, in one sense, a kind of time (though it is not by Plotinus called 'time', *chronos*) that is *not* dependent on or intertwined with human experience, namely eternity (*aiōn*). Indeed, the relationship of time to eternity is, for Plotinus, closely parallel to the relationship of Soul, or of experience bound up inextricably with the physical cosmos, to that of the Intellect, the noetic realm of which that cosmos is a copy.[5]

---

4 The view is attributed to other commentators as an interpretation of Plato by Simplicius, *On Aristotle's Physics* 4.10, 700,16–22 Diels and 705,3–7 Diels. The view of the second-century Platonist Plutarch is that time is 'motion in an orderly fashion that involves measure and limits and revolutions' (*Platonic Questions* 8.4, 1007c–d).
5 I simplify here drastically. Whether, for Plato and his successors (and for Parmenides before him), eternity should be understood as a sort of time, namely time of endless duration – an infinity of time – or rather as timelessness, is problematic and debated; see Sorabji (1983): 98–130. What is clear, at least, for Plotinus and other Neoplatonists, is that the nature and the experience of time and of eternity are fundamentally different in nature, that the highest life for Plotinus involves a move away from the mode of existence entailed by time and (back) to that involved in eternity. The question arises, whether or not it is actually *we* who can have experience of the latter, which belongs to the 'higher' realm, above or beyond the individuation and physicality involved in human souls or selves. On the experiential aspect of Plotinus' account see Sorabji (1983): 157–63 and, in much more detail, Tempest-Walters (2020).

We have followed a train of thought from Plato to the later Platonic tradition; let us now move back to Plato's immediate successor, Aristotle, and briefly consider his hugely influential discussion of time in the *Physics*.[6] As already observed, Aristotle takes it that amongst his own contemporaries some view of time as a form of motion is the standard one. He states that time has been 'usually supposed to be motion and a kind of change'; and it seems likely that in the generations immediately following, the early Stoics, too, subscribed to some version of this 'universally supposed' account: the view is attributed to them that time is 'the interval of motion'.[7]

Both the themes highlighted so far in our overview of philosophical views of time – the relationship with change or motion and the relationship with the human observer – are central to Aristotle's analysis. In summation of the former relationship, Aristotle argues that time is *not* itself a kind of motion or change, but is nevertheless inseparable from, or inconceivable without, change. It 'does not exist without change' (*Physics* 4.11, 218b21), or 'without motion and change' (218b33–219a1); 'time is not a motion, nor is it without motion' (219a1–2). The definitional formula settled upon is the following: 'time is a number of change with respect to the before and after' (219b1–2).

I draw attention to two points in particular. The first is the grounds for the insistence on the inseparability, or inextricability, of time and motion. One motivation seems to be that our awareness of time is inextricable from our awareness of change or motion: we can only discern the passing of time through some perception we have of change taking place within that time. Here, Aristotle talks of the 'motion in the mind' by which we know that time has elapsed.[8] Secondly, in order for the above definition to be meaningful, 'before' and 'after' must be understood as taking their primary sense from something other than time. That is, if 'before' and 'after' are simply identical in meaning to 'earlier in time' and 'later in time', respectively, then the above definition comes out as: 'time is a number of change with respect to what is earlier in time and later in time' – which clearly involves a circularity. Aristotle does, indeed, distinguish different senses of 'before' and 'after' (which could also be translated 'prior' and 'posterior'), and his view seems to be that the primary conceptual applica-

---

6 For philosophical analysis of Aristotle's account see especially Coope (2005).
7 Aristotle, *Physics* 4.10, 218b9–b9–10; for the Stoics, SVF 1.93; 2.509; 2.510 and 2.515.
8 'We perceive motion and time simultaneously; for even if it is dark and we are undergoing no bodily experience, but there is some motion in our mind (*psychē*), we are immediately aware that some time has elapsed', *Physics* 4.11, 219a3–6.

tion of the terms is to magnitude, from which follows that to place, and then that to time.[9]

Aristotle raises some different questions, too: for example, the relationship of time to number; the question, whether it is continuous or atomic in its structure, with the related problem of its theoretically infinite divisibility, as related to our perception of moments of time; the paradox of the 'ceasing instant', or of how it is that the present becomes the past, or how one is to conceptualize the boundary between them.

A large volume of scholarship has been devoted to the elucidation of the considerable intricacies of Aristotle's discussion, and to the question of its coherence or persuasiveness, and it is beyond my scope to engage with that scholarship in detail here. The above account of certain crucial points of Aristotle's analysis, and of the problems that they raise for the later tradition to grapple with, will suffice for the purposes of our further investigations, which will focus on the response given by Galen to this Aristotelian account; on Galen's own account of the relationship between time and motion, and between both and the human observer; and on the significance of these questions for the medical discourse.

Before turning to that response and that further discussion, however, it will be helpful to conclude our scene-setting with a brief summary of two further sets of time-related sources and discussions, namely those focussed on atomism or the atomic structure of time, on the one hand, and those concerned with the (in some ways closely related) analysis of time units and rhythms, in musical theory, on the other.

Aristotle favours the view that time, like the physical universe, is continuous in its structure, and he attributes to the proponents of atomic theory an atomism not just of matter, but also of time, taking the one kind of atomism to be entailed by the other.[10] Beyond Aristotle's evidence, we also have testimony for the notion of atomic or indivisible units of time – again in conjunction with an analogous conception of matter – being espoused by Diodorus Cronus.[11]

---

9 Further on the structure of Aristotle's arguments on the priority of 'before and after' in motion, and space, to that in time, see Coope (2005: 47–81), identifying as a central motivation the claim to explain temporal asymmetry on the model of the parallel asymmetry, or ordered nature, of the other two. A vindication of Aristotle's views in general, and of the coherence of his account of this relationship in particular, is attempted by Detel (forthcoming).
10 See *Physics* 6.1, 231b18–20: 'It is logically the same thing for magnitude, time and motion to be composed of indivisibles, and to be divided into indivisibles or into nothing.'
11 The most relevant text is Sextus Empiricus, *Against the Mathematicians* 10.119–20, where the language used is that of the 'unparted' or 'partless' (*amerēs*) (though some scholars have doubt-

A connection may be drawn between this analysis of time within the Atomist tradition and an account of rhythm which is found in a technical work of music theory. The fourth-century Aristotelian music theorist Aristoxenus of Tarentum developed a theory of rhythm based on a notion of 'rhythmizables' (*rhuthmizomena*), that is, domains that admit of temporal analysis or division,[12] and here he proposed the notion of 'primary times' or 'primary time units' (*prōtoi chronoi*), that is, of minimal units of time which admit of no further division.

Both the further interpretation of this scheme and its relevance to the theoretical and practical discussions of time and speed measurement found in medical writing constitute complex questions, to which we shall return.

For the moment, let this brief summary suffice by way of pointing to the most relevant elements of the theoretical background, in both philosophical and musical discussions. We shall proceed to consider in more detail the views of Galen, of both a philosophical/theoretical nature and of a more practical and clinically-oriented nature; and in the latter context we shall contextualize his approach and his analysis in its relationship with the previous medical, and also musical, discourse.

Galen on time (1): evidence for his theoretical analysis

Let us then consider Galen's 'fragmentary' remarks on the nature of time, that is, those attributed to him by later authors, and apparently deriving from his lost work of logical theory and method, *Demonstration*. The texts in question are brief, and isolated from their original context; and they consist of a mixture of indirect attributions and verbatim quotations. They are relayed by hostile witnesses, the Aristotelian commentators Themistius and Simplicius, who offer a cursory reconstruction of the Galenic argument against Aristotle in order to refute it, and who are writing roughly two and four centuries after the time of Galen, respectively, as well as possibly introducing their own distortions and their own terminology. The text of Simplicius, moreover, is at least partially copied from the text of Themistius. From the point of view of the scholar trying to reconstruct an author's original argument or meaning, therefore, these texts

---

ed whether this language should be taken to imply an atomic view of time; on this issue see Sorabji 1983: 19–20). For a summary of the evidence for and scholarship on Diodorus, see Sedley (2009); and see further Sedley (1977); Denyer (1981), (2009).

12 On Aristoxenus see Barker (1978), (2005); Litchfield (1988); Pearson (1990), West (1992), Gibson (2005). On the relevance of Aristoxenus to the medical discourse, as further discussed below, see Berrey (2017).

manifest some highly problematic features; they also await systematic analysis in the context of Galen's thought.[13] Nevertheless, it seems that something of interest can be gleaned from them.

In the interests of clarity, I offer a brief summary of what I believe that something to be, before laying out the most relevant of these texts for closer inspection.

Galen parts company with Aristotle on the relationship of time and motion, and on the nature of our perception of them. As outlined above, Aristotle says that the perception of time is in some sense only possible because of motion, and that our understanding of before and after in time is dependent on the *spatial* notion of before and after. Galen apparently counter-argues that the perception of time is *sui generis* – that time can only be defined in its own terms and that it is not true that our perception of it is inextricable from that of motion. In this context, then, Galen also denies that the spatial concept of 'before and after' can be transferred to the assessment of time. He thus perhaps accuses Aristotle of precisely the circularity mentioned above. For if 'before' and 'after' have a specific meaning in relation to time, and their use in application to time can only be understood in relation to this specific meaning, and not on analogy with or by transfer from a spatial conception, then a definition of time in terms of 'the before and after' is simply a definition of time in terms of time.[14]

Here is the first testimony, which comes from Themistius' commentary on (and justification of the views expressed in) that central discussion in Aristotle's *Physics*.

> One should pay no attention to Galen, who holds that time is defined through itself. For, having given a detailed enumeration of the many meanings of the before and after, he states that none is applicable to the definition [of time] except the one with respect to time, so that time is 'the number of motion with respect to time'. But it must be understood that the before and the after in motion are not respectively before and after because of time … it comes about from that in relation to magnitude and position, with which it is continuous. Aristotle states this explicitly too: 'The before and after in place is primary; this is

---

13 Such analysis will be provided by Sean Coughlin, Matyáš Havrda and Pauline Koetschet, who are working on an edition of Galen's fragmentary *Demonstration* on the basis of all the testimonia. My remarks and summary analysis here are, by contrast, highly provisional. I am extremely grateful to Sean Coughlin for drawing my attention to these texts, and for personal communications related to them.
14 It could be argued, conversely, that he embraces this circularity, as it were on Aristotle's behalf, since his claim is indeed that time can only be understood in terms of time, that only the temporal sense of 'before' and 'after' is applicable to it. At any rate it seems he must argue that *if* one accepts Aristotle's definition of time, one must accept the circularity; he is attacking the move by which Aristotle transfers the spatial sense of 'before' and 'after' to the temporal one.

where it is in position; but since it is also in magnitude, it is necessarily also in motion' [219a14–17]. Still, even if it be granted that the before and after in motion mean nothing other than the before and after in time, as he thinks, what problem arises from that?[15]

The second passage is taken from a little earlier in the same text.

> Evidently, then, time is not without motion – but not in the manner of Galen's interpretation, that is, because it is when in motion that we conceive of time: that is what he takes Aristotle to be saying here. Rather, it is because the notion of time is inextricably linked to that of motion. Why, then, did Galen pointlessly contest this, and produce arguments against it, as follows? 'After all,' he says, 'we also have a conception of immovable things while ourselves being moved – such things as the poles, or the centre of the earth, and these things are not "with motion".' He should have paid attention to where Aristotle explicitly says 'for we perceive time and motion simultaneously'. It makes a very great difference whether we take it that time [has] something of motion on the grounds that [its conception] is inextricably linked to the conception of motion, or on the grounds that it is while in motion that we conceive of time. But this fellow is like this in many contexts.[16]

We move to the first of the passage from Simplicius.

> On the basis of these statements the remarkable Galen, in the eighth book of his *Demonstration*, supposes that Aristotle is stating that time is not without motion on the following grounds, namely that it is when in motion[17] that we conceive of it; here he introduces to the argument the supposed absurdity that completely unmoved bodies would have to be 'with motion', since our conception of them too is 'with motion', for we do not conceive of anything while our conception is devoid of motion. He might equally say on these grounds that unextended things could not be without extension, since we conceive of them with extension (acting for the most part through the imagination).[18]

Here, the interpretation is attributed to Galen that by 'time is not without motion' Aristotle means that we, the subjects or perceivers of time, are in motion at any point at which we conceive or conceptualize it; if there were no more to the argument than this, then, *everything* which we conceptualize would have to be conceptualized as involving motion, since we are ourselves never at rest.

A little further on Simplicius produces further anti-Galenic arguments, partially overlapping with those of the first passage from Themistius above, while also introducing some new material.

---

15 Themistius, *On Aristotle's Physics*, 4.11 (149,4–19 Schenkl).
16 Themistius, *On Aristotle's Physics* 4.11 (144,23–145,2 Schenkl).
17 Reading κινούμενοι (i.e., 'when *we* are in motion') for κινούμενον ('when *it* is in motion'), as seems required by comparison with the summary of the same argument above in the Themistius text.
18 Simplicius, *On Aristotle's Physics* 4.11 (708,27–34 Diels)

Since the most learned Galen argued against some of these statements, saying that time is made evident through itself, let us present his argument for discussion. [*There follows, almost verbatim, the second sentence of the first Themistius passage above, and then Themistius' counter-argument (with explicit attribution to him), from 'But it must be understood' to 'also in motion'.*]

To this Galen might respond that the before and after in motion is consequent upon that in magnitude, for it is in this context that motion, in terms of before and after, is especially in relation to place: that is what it is to be before and after in magnitude. But that the before with respect to time, as already stated, is something else, which accompanies the motion in terms of before and after, but does not possess before and after in place, but in the extension of being, this being something distinct from that in terms of place, which comes about through motion.

Themistius introduces a second solution, too: [*there follows the passage from the first Themistius passage above: 'Still, even if it be granted', etc. ...*]

Galen might respond to this, too, as follows: that if the before and after in motion were the same thing as the before and after in time, then the statement that time was the before and after in motion would be sound, and in that case time would not be made evident through itself. If, however, that with respect to place is one thing, which is not temporal, while that with respect to time is another, then one would have to state that time is the before and after in motion with respect to time. Perhaps, then, one must understand the before and after in terms of the extension of being, not in terms of place, and so time is signified through itself. And its name, then, will not be, in straightforward terms, the same as 'the before and the after', but the same as a particular kind of before and after; and this is the definition.[19]

There is a certain amount here that is not clear, both in the counter-arguments to Aristotle attributed to Galen and in the refutations of these by Themistius and Simplicius. There is, too, one specific problem of interpretation, arising from a point in the text which otherwise might be thought to be the most helpful in elucidating Galen's position. We feel the need of some further elaboration of the bald statement attributed to Galen of the self-revealing nature of time, that it is understood only in its own terms or 'made evident' through itself; and here Simplicius' suggestion that Galen's motion-independent understanding of time may be further understood in terms of the 'extension of being' (*hē tou einai paratasis*) might be thought fruitful. Unfortunately, however, it seems that it must be distrusted, as it turns out that the phrase in question is one beloved of Simplicius, but very little attested elsewhere in Greek literature. The conclusion that it

---

19 Simplicius, *On Aristotle's Physics* 4.11 (718,13–719,18 Diels)

is Simplicius' own gloss, rather than a further quotation from Galen, seems unavoidable.[20]

In spite of these problems, however, and of the dimness with which Galen's original argument can be discerned through the murky thickets of a problematic textual tradition and hostile later scholarship, his attack on the Aristotelian definition, and the fundamental position attributed to him, of time as something only perceptible or measurable in its own terms, not by reference to place or magnitude, seems a distinctive and noteworthy one.

It should be added that there is a further piece of evidence that Galen argued for the conceptual independence of time and motion. Such a view is attributed to him by a tenth-century Arabic author, Ibn Abī Saʿīd:[21]

> Galen's view was that time is eternal, and does not need motion to exist; and he states that Plato was of a like opinion on this point. That is to say that he considered that time is a substance, meaning by that duration, and that motion measures it. Galen states accordingly that motion does not produce time for us; it only produces for us days, months and years. Time, on the other hand, exists *per se*, and is [not] an accident consequent on motion.

Sorabji doubted the reliability of this testimony, preferring the view that Galen held that time could exist without *orderly celestial* motion, but not without motion altogether. However, there seems to be no explicit evidence associating Galen with that narrower view; and, more importantly, the view ascribed to him by Ibn Abī Saʿīd seems to accord perfectly with that which has emerged, albeit dimly, from our other evidence.

Galen on time (2): further analysis and justification

If, then, we have established Galen's theoretical position in broad outline, a little more should be said by way of elucidation of this position, as well as of its likely motivation and justification.

For the above passages from Themistius and Simplicius raise a rather obvious question, to which we may be keen to determine the answer. Is Galen grossly misunderstanding Aristotle, as Themistius impatiently suggests, or is Themistius failing to grasp Galen's legitimate objection and alternative point of view? In

---

20 The terminology perhaps finds a parallel in Augustine's understanding of time as an extension, in particular an extension of the mind (*Confessions* 11.26), discussed by Sorabji (1983): 30–1.

21 I here give the most relevant part of the text here, which was published by Pines (1955), to whom the translation is due, and discussed by Sorabji (1983): 82–3.

what follows, I shall suggest that Galen's view at least deserved something better than the Aristotelian commentator's contempt and at best was a reasonable view for which he was able to offer a coherent argument – one, indeed, which we may find persuasive.

Themistius accuses of Galen of reducing Aristotle's statement that 'time is not without motion' to the banal proposition that 'we are always in motion when we perceive time' and then proceeding to argue that this banal proposition can have no force relevant to the point at issue. For, by virtue of the same proposition, we are *always* in motion, also while conceiving of things without motion. Thus, if Aristotle, as Galen claims, relies on this proposition for his view of time, he would by the same token have to argue that 'things without motion are not without motion': we are in motion while we perceive them, too.

So, according to Themistius, Galen has taken Aristotle to intend 'not without motion' to refer to the state of the subject or observer, not to an external object or state observed over a passage of time, and thus plainly to distort Aristotle's intention.

But is Galen's interpretation as crass as Themistius suggests? Or, to turn the question around, in what sense *are* we to take Aristotle's statement that time is not without motion, and might Galen's criticism of his view correspond to a coherent interpretation of it?

Let us say that Aristotle means that we cannot either perceive, or imagine, time passing without also perceiving or imagining some motion which takes place over that time. But any particular observed object, at least, *may* remain completely still during that period; there may be no observable motion. Surely that can be generalized, at least in principle, to the totality of things we observe over a given period of time. It is possible to observe an external state of affairs, at least over a very short period of time, in which no motion at all takes place, or at least one in which we are aware of no motion. (And it is certainly possible to conceive of oneself making such an observation or lack of observation.) There is therefore a clear conceptual separation; there can be periods of time which pass without observable motion. (We might, indeed, wish to say that the very fact that there can be *more or less* motion itself is sufficient to establish the conceptual separation.)

The counter-argument will presumably go roughly as follows. We are, nonetheless, constantly aware of some motion – if not of change as observed in the outside world, then at least of our own breathing or heartbeat. Well, Galen could say, these too could theoretically be stopped, at least for a short period. Perhaps, then, a *mental* motion is sufficient. This, perhaps, is the point on which Aristotle may be taken to rely. As we observed, he speaks (at *Physics* 219a4–7) of such a 'motion of the mind' in justification of his view. The passing of time, then, the

Aristotle/Themistius argument goes, is only observed because something happens – a mental activity, which may be defined as a motion – and we measure or perceive time against that.

Against this, Galen's argument could reasonably take one (or both) of two tacks. First, to point out that the mental motion, too, is only contingently present: just like any observed external motion, it can be present more or less. Our argument in relation to external motions was that they may be absent, or so little present as not to be observed, and that therefore our perception of the passage of time cannot be taken to depend on them. But internal 'motions', of our body or mind, too, may be present to a greater or lesser extent, while the same amount of time passes; how then can we define time as inseparable from this kind of motion, any more than from the other?

Or (the second tack): why should we define the mental activity by which we have consciousness of time passing as a 'motion'? That is: we can imagine a mental state in which we are conscious of no motion – in the standardly accepted, spatial, sense – not even an internal motion 'of the mind'; but we would still be conscious of the passing of time. Of course, it is open to Aristotle to claim – and indeed he apparently does claim – that such mental consciousness of time passing is, indeed, a motion. But Galen might, surely, be justified in demanding some further argument in support of that claim. And, in the absence of any such further argument, in holding to a view that such mental awareness of the passing of time is not, itself, a motion.

Does it not, then, make sense to regard this mental awareness of the passage of time – so long as we have been given no good grounds for subsuming it under the heading of 'motion' – as corresponding to something that is definable in its own terms, and *not* in the same terms as those of motion – to state that it is 'made evident by itself', separate in kind from motion? To look at it the other way round: what justification is there for taking space or motion as the prior category, and regarding our perception of time as some derivative of it?

It seems to me that it is plausible that Galen's argument could have taken some such form as the above, even if not expressed in precisely those terms. It seems to me, further, that an argument along those lines is a convincing one, in leading to the conclusion that perception of time and that of motion are *not*, indeed, inseparable – or at the very least in casting doubt on that conceptual inseparability.

We have then an account of why Galen might – in my view, with reasonable justification – have asserted that time was 'made manifest only by itself'. In terms of the further structure of his lost argument, then, we can understand how on that basis he could have proceeded to an attempted *reductio* of Aristotle's position along the lines that 'we are always in motion when we think of motionless bodies too'. It is, in Galen's view, Aristotle who is guilty of the confusion, because it can only be, on the best possible account of his theory, some motion internal to us which establishes that time is always with motion. But such internal motion may or not be present, or at least it may be present to a greater or lesser extent; its presence is therefore contingent and cannot be an intrinsic feature of time's passing. Since, then, the two are conceptually separate, and any motion going on within us is not directly or essentially related to the passing of time, Galen's *reductio* hits the mark. It is, of course, completely irrelevant to our mental conception of a motionless body that our own body happens to be in motion while we have that conception. But, as Galen's argument shows, precisely the same irrelevance applies in the case of time and motion, since *all that Aristotle can coherently be taken to mean* by 'time is not without motion' is indeed that there will, generally, be some motion going on while we perceive. That motion, on Galen's view, is just as irrelevant to the conception in the one case as in the other.

Whether or not we find Galen's view persuasive, however, it seems to have found few advocates within the ancient philosophical tradition. A partial parallel is perhaps found in Augustine, who, in an argument against the view that times are celestial motions, made the point that time would not be affected if the heavenly bodies either stood still or were accelerated; elsewhere, however, he does seem explicitly to accept the dependence of time upon change.[22]

On a broader perspective, Galen's view seems to find an echo in the modern 'substantivist' or 'absolutist' view, in philosophy and physics, according to which time is conceptually independent of those things which happen within time. In the early modern period, such a view is associated with Isaac Newton, and sometimes called the 'empty time' or 'bucket' view.[23] A more recent philosophical attempt to justify the notion that the passing of time does not necessarily involve change was made by Shoemaker.[24] It may be said that neither this nor the 'empty' view have been found widely persuasive in contemporary philosophy

---

22 *Confessions* 11.23; 12.8 and 11; *City of God* 11.6 and 12.16. The passages and Augustine's view are discussed by Sorabji (1983): 30–1.

23 It is also sometimes referred to as 'Platonism with respect to time', although, as has already emerged, this term is misleading. The attribution of such a view to Plato is, at least, disputed within the Platonic tradition: see n. 4 above.

24 See Shoemaker (1969); also Newton-Smith (1980), arguing for the possibility of 'empty time' but against the absolutist view. For an overview of philosophical views that time does or does not involve change, see Emery et al. (2020), section 2, with further literature cited there. Relevant to the ancient, including Galen's, discussions of the fundamental nature of time *perception* is also Prosser (2016).

or physics, which rather emphasizes the fundamental inextricability of space and time.[25]

Galen on speed: the measurement of the pulse

We move to a more practical area, although here too we shall consider Galenic, and other medical, analyses of a theoretical nature, regarding both time and its relationship with motion.[26]

Galen's discussion of our perception of speed arises in the context of the medical assessment of the speed of the pulse. Here, as before, some filling-in of the complex theoretical background will be needed before we proceed further – in this case, the theoretical background concerning the discernible distinctions within the motions of the pulse, which were taken to be of great clinical importance.

Galen identifies five key variables in relation to the pulse: speed, size, tension, hardness or softness of the artery wall, contents of the artery ('fulness' or 'emptiness').[27] Two further complexities, or sets of variables, must however be added. One set arises from the internal relationship of the different parts of the pulse: 'in all these respects ... there will sometimes be evenness, and sometimes unevenness; and there will be some ratio of the time of the expansion (*diastolē*) and that of the contraction (*systolē*)'. (For fuller explanation of Galen's physical theory of the *diastolē* and *systolē* see below, p. 141 with n. 33.)

---

25 But the absolutist view of *both* space and time, i.e. the view of their existence independent of their contents, does form part of a debate in modern science; see Mitchell (1993).
26 On Galen's theory and practice in relation to the pulse see Barton (1994a), Lewis (2016); and for a broader, comparative perspective Kuriyama (1999). On the Galenic physiological background see Harris (1973), and for the most relevant pre-Galenic history of pulse theory see Lewis (2017) (on Praxagoras), von Staden (1989) and Berrey (2017) (on Herophilus).
27 Galen presents the different sets of variables in a number of subtly, and sometimes confusingly, different ways; and in particular he sometimes casts doubt on the validity of the category of 'fulness'; on these issues see Lewis (2022), (forthcoming). My summary here is based primarily on *The Distinct Types of Pulse* 1.3 (VIII.500–1 K.): 'There must, then, quite necessarily be [1] some time of these motions ... as well as some time specific to the periods of rest. Since the artery possesses three dimensions ... length, breadth and depth, it is absolutely necessary that there be [2] some quantity in each of the dimensions, both of expansion and of contraction. It is also necessary that it be in [3] some state of tension, so that it is acting either with difficulty and feebly, or readily and vigorously; and that [4] the actual tunic of the artery be soft or hard, but also [5] the internal breadth be as it were empty or full.'

For our purposes this last-mentioned 'ratio' is of particular importance. The ratio between the two phases of the pulse, also known as the rhythm, is a crucial, and contested, diagnostic concept. In fact, there are, on a more precise analysis, *four* phases in the pulse: the expansion (E), the period of rest which follows the expansion before the commencement of the contraction (R1), the contraction (C), and the period of rest which follows the contraction before the commencement of the next expansion (R2). On this analysis, then, the ratio or rhythm will we that of E + R1 to C + R2. (This more precise analysis has another important consequence, as we shall see shortly.)

We have, then, covered all the distinctions that can arise – but only those which can arise *within any one beat* of the pulse. There remains a final set of variables.

For there are two other, 'systematic' distinctions, as they are known, whereby we consider the evenness and unevenness and the regularity and irregularity of a number of pulses compared with each other.[28]

These last two terms, then, 'unevenness' and 'irregularity', pick out discrepancies between the manifestation of one or more of the above variables in the first beat with their manifestation in the next, or later, beats.

Now there is something very striking that emerges here, especially if we wish to consider the Galenic project of pulse diagnosis in relation to its modern descendant. For under neither of the two broad headings – that of variables discernible within a single beat or that of variables discernible over a series of successive ones – has Galen mentioned the one variable in the pulse which is standardly assessed today: the rate of the pulse. Is this because pulse rate plays no part in his system? Yes and no. In fact, the conception of *puknotēs* – that is, how frequent, or how 'close together', the successive beats of the pulse are – did play an essential role in pulse diagnosis, for both Galen and other ancient medical practitioners (as we shall see shortly).[29] That sounds

---

28 See further the text cited on p. 142.
29 When used in a temporal context, *puknotēs* could reasonably translated as 'frequency', in the sense of how often something occurs in a given time. In view of the difficulty, which I here outline, in equating the notion with that of 'rate' of the pulse, and the additional complication that 'frequency' in modern-day medicine has a separate, technical meaning in relation to the pulse, I for the moment preserve the word in transliterated form. 'Closeness' or 'density' provides a good approximation to the core sense of the term, which in Greek usually has a spatial reference, and is less commonly applied to time intervals. It is noteworthy that Galen himself claims that the fundamental sense of the opposed terms *araios* and *puknos* is that of porousness and the lack of it: something is *araios* if it is 'run through with large channels', and *puknos* if its 'run through with small ones', i.e. dense. It is from this physical sense, says Galen, that the others, including temporal frequency or scarcity, are derived (see *Health* 2.5, 53–4 Koch, VI.119 K.).

very like the conception of pulse rate; it seems that it should yield the same result. In fact, however, the two conceptions are, for Galen at least, significantly different. Moreover, the difference is important and instructive.

Galen makes the clear distinction, just outlined, between differences discerned within one beat and those discerned over several. Yet he does not mention *puknotēs* – how close the beats are together – in the latter category. *Puknotēs* does appear; but it appears as a subcategory amongst the variables discernible within one beat. Specifically, it is a subcategory within the first such variable, namely 'time', i.e. the duration and speed of that single beat's motion (or of the parts of its motion). Yet surely *puknotēs* – how close or frequent the beats are – is, by definition, a function of the relationship between successive beats? How, then, does Galen's apparently illogical and nonsensical categorization of it come about?

The explanation is in fact quite straightforward.[30] On the most precise analysis, as we have seen, there are four phases of the pulse: the *diastolē* or expansion (E), the period of rest after the expansion (R1), the *systolē* or contraction (C), and the period of rest after contraction (R2). For Galen, the duration of each of these can and must be considered separately; and each is in principle measurable (albeit not, as we shall see, with complete precision).

Galen defines *puknotēs* in terms of the length, or shortness, of the interval between the end of one pulse and the beginning of the next. It is, indeed, the 'closeness' of one pulse beat to the next, understood in terms of the shortness of that interval between one end and the next beginning – that is, R2. We, by contrast, measure pulse rate in terms of a number of beats per minute; here the relevant interval must be that between the beats themselves, or more precisely between the precisely equivalent moment within each beat. Take a rate of 80 beats per minute: the relevant individual timespan is 0.75 seconds: that is, this is the length of time that elapses, on average, between one beat and the next, or to be precise between the equivalent moments within those two beats. Now, it might be thought that the difference between measuring the time between the equivalent moments within two successive beats, and measuring the time of the interval between the end of one and the beginning of the next, was trivial. In fact, it is of considerable significance.

On Galen's model, as we have seen, each individual pulse consists of four phases: E, R1, C, R2. Each element within that may be longer or shorter. It

---

[30] For Galen's account of the fact (which he acknowledges is not universally agreed) that *puknotēs*, although in a sense a feature of a set taken together, is indeed discernible within one beat, see *The Distinct Types of Pulse* 1.6 (VIII.511 K.).

would thus, in principle, be possible for an E of very long duration, or an E + R1 + C of very long joint duration, to be combined with an R2 of very short duration. Conversely, the whole of the E + R1 + C might be completed exceptionally quickly, while R2 was unusually long. It will thus be readily seen that length of R2 cannot possibly be used to give a measurement that would equate to pulse rate. It could happen that the beats were *puknoi* – 'close' – in Galen's sense, but that the total number over a minute turned out to be unusually low. Conversely, a case where the beats were the opposite of *puknoi* (*araioi*, 'spaced out'), i.e., where R2 was quite long, would give a high reading per minute if the other phases, E + R1 + C, were exceptionally fast.

We shall turn to the question of the measurement of *puknotēs* – in fact, the only of these variables for which there is ancient evidence of some kind of *quantitative* project of measurement, using observer-independent apparatus – towards the end of the chapter.

For now, let us note a crucial conceptual point which has emerged from the above. Galen neither singles out 'rate', in the way that we would expect any clinical observer of the pulse to do, nor, in fact, does he have a distinct class of 'rate', separate from his observation of a single beat of the pulse. The result is striking. At one level, it is a function of a technical or semantic difference, in his definition of terms: he is able to subsume *puknotēs*, the variable corresponding to how frequently the beats recur, under the heading of length of time taken up by the rest at the end of the pulse beat. On another, it bespeaks a fundamental difference in scientific model and expectation. The problem or omission we perceive here – namely that there is nothing, on this model, that corresponds to our beats per minute – simply does not occur to Galen. It is no part of his project or ambition to give a quantitative measurement of the time periods in question, something which can only be achieved through such measurement of time over a longer period such as a minute, followed by division of the result of that measurement. Thus, for his purposes, the definition of pulse rate – or more precisely, of the 'closeness' between beats – in terms of the smallness of the interval between the end of one and the beginning of the next makes perfect sense, and leads to no conceptual oddity or problem.

Let us, then, leave both pulse rate and *puknotēs* to one side, and return to the first and fundamental set of differentiae mentioned above – those assessed within one beat. What does it actually mean to measure the *speed*, as opposed to the frequency, of a pulse? In general terms, Galen is clear what is meant by the speed of any object. It is understood – uncontroversially enough – in terms of the relationship between distance traversed and the time in which it is traversed. Galen gives a number of examples involving people traversing distances measured in *stadia*.

> Let us take it that there are two motions, one of which completes fifty *stadia* in one hour, the other 150 *stadia* in three hours. Should we, then, also say that these are equal in speed? Of course we should. ... Motions which cover an equal distance in an equal time will be equal in speed. ... If, on the other hand, the ratio of distance to distance is greater than that of time to time, or that of time to time greater than that of distance to distance, then we shall no longer consider the motions equal in speed. ... Let us say that there is one motion covering a distance of 400 cubits and another one of 100, while the time is two hours in the former case and one hour in the latter. ... Evidently if we imagine the former motion covering only the 100 cubits, it will do so within half an hour. It will thus be swifter than the second motion, since it covers an equal distance in a shorter time. If, meanwhile, we conceive of the second motion covering the 400 cubits, it will require four hours to do so, and so will be slower than the former motion, since it covers an equal distance in a longer time.[31]

Galen is never averse from labouring a point, and the above (abridged) account seems to make one which is simple enough – that both distance and time need to be known in order to assess speed – in a very painstaking and even roundabout way. Galen's laborious and circuitous examples, however, remind us of an important feature of such measurements in the ancient world. Longer units, both of distance and of time, are much more readily measured, in everyday life, than shorter ones. In the case of time, as was already observed in our first chapter, units shorter than an hour are problematic; in terms of distances, too, those most easily measurable will be the larger-scale ones, known or marked out in or between public spaces. This is not a world of readily accessible or portable instruments of measurement, of either distance or time. One result of this is that calculations of relative speed will tend to proceed on the basis of the kind of processes of division or multiplication of known or readily observable units outlined in this passage. In fact, nothing is being said, here, about the instruments by which these measurements are made; but the everyday examples Galen gives rely on a scale of measurement – in time, hours; in distance, longer units – that would be publicly available and accessible.

But the point of producing these examples is, for Galen, precisely to address the challenge of the measurement of the speed of the pulse. In principle, exactly the same applies here as there: one should know the distance covered and the length of time in which it is covered.[32] So, again, the motion of what, and

---

[31] *The Discernment of the Pulse* 2.1 (VIII.830–3 K.).
[32] The point is made explicitly: 'If we already know how great a distance the well-balanced pulse accomplishes in how long a time, and then in the case of another pulse, which has the same time, we find a shorter distance, we will say that the latter has been moved during a long time period ... we shall say that a pulse which happens in a short time is quick and one that happens in a long time is slow,' *The Discernment of the Pulse* 3.1 (VIII.880 K.).

over what distance, is being measured when we measure the speed of a pulse? In order to answer this, we need to understand in a little more detail the Galenic conception of the motion of the pulse itself. Galen takes the arterial motion of the pulse to consist in a vehement outward motion or expansion of the artery – the *diastolē* or expansion – followed by a return or inward motion, the *systolē* or contraction.[33] In the course of the outward motion or expansion, the artery is extended in three dimensions, and each of them – height (or depth), length and breadth – is potentially significant. And the amount of this extension is the *size* (*megethos*). The second variable is the forcefulness or vehemence (*sphodrotēs*) of the observed impact. The third is the speed. Speed must not, as already mentioned, be confused with 'closeness', *puknotēs*, on the one hand; nor do increases in speed go along with those in size, on the other. A *puknos* ('close' or 'frequent') pulse – not a *fast* pulse – is one in which successive beats occur close to each other in time. Two pulses may have exactly the same *puknotēs* and they may, further, have exactly the same size – that is, the point of maximum extension of the artery may be the same. But this point of maximum extension, as well as the return to the minimum extension, may be arrived at twice as fast in the one case as the other: this will be a difference in speed.

What has to be measured, then, in a measurement of the speed of the pulse is the time taken for the artery to reach that maximum extension, considered in relation to the distance moved by it in the course of that motion. The time and distance taken in its return to the unexpanded state may similarly be measured.[34] There is a period of rest, after both *diastolē* and *systolē*, which however

---

[33] The terminology is potentially confusing in relation to modern medical usage, where 'systolic' and 'diastolic' refer to motions of the heart, the former motion – that is, the contraction of the heart valves – corresponding to the pumping of blood, the latter being the period of its relaxation and refilling with blood. In ancient pulse theory, by contrast, what is at issue is a motion of the *artery*, rather than the heart, and *diastolē* and *systolē* refer, respectively, to the artery's expansion and contraction. The *diastolē* is the outward (in our terms, pumping) motion, the *systolē* the relaxation or contraction, *of the artery*; and thus the sense of the two terms – as regards the phases to which they refer – is effectively reversed, in relation to our usage. In what follows, I shall continue to use 'expansion' for *diastolē* and 'contraction' for *systolē*.

[34] In fact, there is lengthy Galenic discussion of the role of the *systolē* or contraction in pulse assessment: this was a controversial question in the tradition on the pulse, with Herophilus and Archigenes asserting that it *was* perceptible and others, especially the Empiricists, denying it. Galen's view is that while the *systolē* is perceptible, its perception and accurate discernment are performed only at a highly advanced stage of clinical practice, and are not available to all, not even to all doctors. (See e.g. *The Pulse for Beginners* 4, VIII.456–7 K.; *The Discernment of the Pulse* 1.1, VIII.770–1 K.) One may thus for certain purposes operate according to a simplified system in which one takes into account only the *diastolē*.

should not be taken into account, as what is to be assessed is the speed of the actual motion.

We are now reasonably clear, at least, what it is that is being measured, and what facts need to be discovered in order for such a measurement to made. But here we immediately come up against a problem, that of the technology or methodology involved: how, in practice, is any such measurement performed?

In fact, no non-human apparatus is relevant, from Galen's point of view. The technology of measurement is rather the human perceptual apparatus – in the context of the pulse, that is the sense of touch – which, however, can be brought by training to a high level of perceptiveness, discerning degrees of difference and indeed actual phenomena which to begin with are completely imperceptible. It will be worth offering a quotation from Galen's vivid and enthusiastic account of the development of such perceptual and analytical skills; the following passage also lists succinctly the range of detectable variables in Galen's scheme (already summarized above):

> Sculptors and painters train their optical sense, wine-makers and cooks their sense of taste, those involved in the preparation of scents their sense of smell, and musicians their sense of hearing, not for days or months but for many years in order to achieve the necessary precision – and this in spite of the fact that they have the materials for this practice constantly available to them. How much time, then, should one imagine that a doctor requires for the training of his sense of touch? The doctor has to recognize a very large number ways in which the artery is affected ... first, he must recognize [1] the size of the dimensional extension, then [2] the quality and [3] the time of the motion; then, too, [4] tension of the capacity that moves them, then [5] the condition of the tunic of the artery itself. All these he must recognize simultaneously, during the expansion of the artery ... but the same range also during the contraction – and then there is the period which intervenes between them, while the pulse is at rest (which period is itself dual in nature, consisting of that which follows the expansion and precedes the contraction and that which follows the contraction and precedes the expansion), and the ratio between these two, that of the one period of the motion to the other and that of the one period of rest to the other, as well as that of the composite to the composite. All these must be recognized before the second beat of the artery, as the first pulse is completed. Then, as the second begins, you must examine the same things that were indicated in the first pulse, and compare the findings of that one with those of the present one, in order to identify their evenness or unevenness, and all the distinctions; then, you must consider three, four, five and indeed many successive pulses, in order to know their order or lack of it.
>
> How long a period of practice do you think is needed for this? If I may state my own opinion honestly, I would say that a whole human lifetime is required to achieve perfect knowledge.[35]

---

35 *The Discernment of the Pulse* 1.1 (VIII.768–70 K.).

He continues, via an autobiographical remark about the 'wonderful desire' that he nurtured, from an early age, for the art concerning the pulse, to discuss the debate amongst his predecessors (cf. note 34 above) about the discernibility or not of the *contraction* of the pulse, and his own related confusion. He continues in autobiographical vein:

> I languished in this state of deep uncertainty for a considerable number of years; but I did not abandon the enquiry and, by constant application, I gradually acquired the impression of a contraction clear to the sense of touch. In the course of still further training, then, this ceased to be merely a faint impression; the discernment of the contraction became something as manifest as that of the expansion. Once this was established, it is difficult even to describe the speed with which I attained to the discernment of the remaining items; they followed at once, and from then on appeared quite clearly, as though a bright light had suddenly been shone in the dark. … What happens is that a certain kind of attainment is being nurtured, the growth of which is so gradual and hidden that until it is fully formed it is not even evident whether or not it has begun; when, however, it does achieve completion it suddenly becomes apparent, producing the fruit of all the previous labours all at once – and, if one may use a vulgar expression, with interest repaid. If those who came after me had even a small fraction of my devotion to these matters, which extends even to the attempt to communicate all the sensory experiences in words, then the art of the pulse could be acquired within a shorter period of training.[36]

A passage from another of the pulse treatises is also relevant to this understanding of the development and refinement of perceptual skill. Here too Galen elaborates on the notion of the ever-increasing ability of the trained senses to make relevant distinctions; and here too he makes a parallel with such technical training in another discipline, that of music. (See figure 14.)

> … the well-balanced within each of the classes is single and indivisible; the others admit of a very large number of divisions, which are infinite in their actual nature, for distinctions of degree in every class … must necessarily be infinite in number, but it is not so in our perception of them, which depends rather on our better and worse training, according to which we will be able either to recognize also the small distinctions or only the more prominent ones.
>
> In the case of musical intervals, a musician will be well able to discern not only an interval of a tone or a semi-tone, but even that of a quarter-tone, while the lay person is not able to hear even an interval of two tones.[37] … in the present case, we have given an account of our

---

36 *The Discernment of the Pulse* 1.1 (VIII.771–3 K.).
37 Both these claims are perhaps less surprising in the ancient musical context than they might be to us. Quarter-tones were a feature of one of the standard Greek 'scales', the enharmonic, whose upward movement began with two such intervals. That same scale was then completed (up to the fourth) with the large interval of a ditone, while another of the standard scales, the

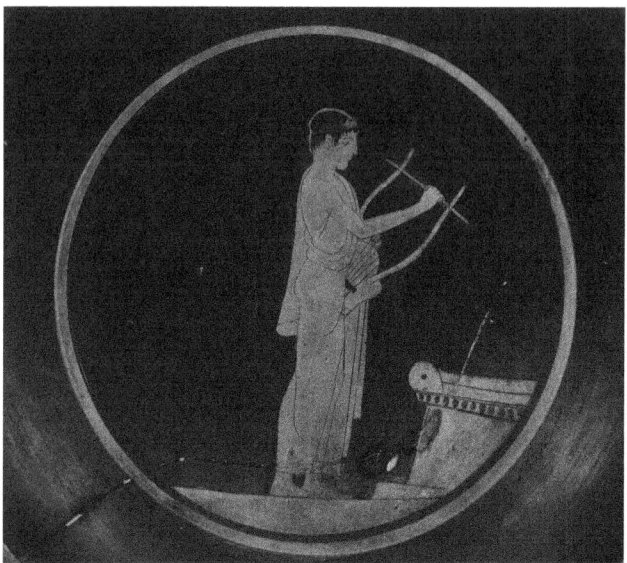

Figure 14: The fine-tuning of the senses (1): tuning a lyre. A youth (captioned as ΚΑΛΟΣ, 'beautiful') is depicted striking strings with his left hand while adjusting pegs with his right. From an Attic red-figure kylix, attributed to the Dish Painter (c. 490–470 BCE), British Museum, 1836,0224.168. Image source: https://www.britishmuseum.org/collection/image/477213001 © The Trustees of the British Museum. Shared under a Creative Commons Attribution-NonCommercial-ShareAlike 4.0 International (CC BY-NC-SA 4.0) licence.

> own perception: we are able to discern six distinctions of pulse by virtue of their excess or deficiency with respect to the well-balanced one, in each class. But it is sufficient for beginners, in the first phase, to perceive one such distinction in each case, and to be able to separate these from the well-balanced one. In the course of time, I suppose, and through practice, they will be able first, perhaps, to make a twofold division, then a threefold one and then a fourfold one.[38]

So, the measurement is one not carried out according to any absolute standard, but in a way relative to the individual perceiver. By the same token, that individ-

---

chromatic, included an interval of a tone-and-a-half. Relatedly, particular intervals, for example the *lichanos* or 'third', existed in many possible versions in different musical contexts, the different possibilities spanning a range of a tone. Thus, while the second of Galen's claims here seems exaggerated, at least for a person with any significant experience of listening to music, it is at least true that in certain contexts a rather wide range of frequencies could be heard as in some sense 'the same note'. (See further n. 56 below, with Aristoxenus' account of such broad pitch ranges.)

38 *The Distinct Types of Pulse* 2.8 (VIII.619–20 K.).

ual may hugely increase his or her capacity to make the relevant distinctions and judgements.

But this still leaves us with a question. For if one is not using any measuring technology, nor attempting the kind of precision that this would involve, there must still be some mental or conceptual standard or scale involved, and this might be of more than one kind. For example, it could be that although not actually checking one's findings against any apparatus, nor aiming to offer any numerical account of those findings, one still has some system of measuring units in mind, of the sort that such an apparatus would provide. Another possibility is that the conceptual measurement is made by reference to no such independent standard at all, the scale being provided rather *internally*, by consideration and experience of the motions of the objects under examination themselves. And this latter alternative seems in fact to be the case.

That is, the observer or practitioner learns to gauge the speed (along with the other variable, size and vehemence) associated with human norms of various sorts – norms for the human species as a whole and, which is more relevant to actual clinical medicine, norms for a particular individual or class of individuals. Further specifications may arise in relation to age, sex, individual constitution, environment, and so on.

Such norms, then, are understood as constituting the relevant midpoint on each of the relevant conceptual scales. 'Large', 'small', 'vehement', 'faint', and so forth, must be understood not as absolute, nor as quantifiable, terms, but as qualitative assessments of a significant departure from that norm or midpoint. It is in virtue of its adherence to or departure from that human midpoint or mean that a mixture or state of the body, a drug, or a particular pulse, is assessed as 'medium' (or 'well-balanced', *summetros*), 'fast', 'slow', and so on. That is what, in such contexts, these terms actually mean. Galen insists on this point, of the relativity of the conception of all such quality terms – specifically, their relativity either to the normal human state in general, or to the normal state of a particular individual – repeatedly, for example in *Mixtures* and in *Simple Drugs* as well as in the pulse treatises. Further refinements can be introduced, on such a conceptual scale; however, they remain qualitative refinements, with no reference to a numerical scale of any kind.

It is noteworthy, indeed, that in the particular context of the pulse Galen actually warns against the ambition to found such judgements on a quantitative basis.

> This [sc. whether a pulse is long or short] cannot be determined by the number of fingers, as is the practice of some, who say that it is long if it extends to four, medium if it extends to three, and short if it extends to two. For there is no single measure of best nature in a body;

it is rather that by starting from one [individual] nature you will easily discover the quantity in each case, providing that you are capable of making an inference to the proportionate quantity. By comparing other human beings with that, you will say, in the case of those with a body of the same overall length, that they have a long or a short pulse. And similarly that they have a pulse which is wide, narrow, high, shallow, or large and small in all three dimensions, for in each case you will judge the others by reference to the point of good balance.[39]

While this may sound terribly vague and subjective, from a contemporary scientific perspective, the ancient medical discourse is remarkable optimistic about what can be discerned by the trained senses – as indeed the above passages make abundantly clear.[40]

There is a further, specific ramification of this, when it comes to the measurement of speed. As we have seen, Galen lays out a clear definition of speed, in terms of distance over time, which seems in theory to correspond to an ambition to give precise measurements of each of these; and indeed, in certain cases, with longer distances and longer time periods, such precise measurements would have been perfectly available to him. When it comes to assessment of speed over very short time periods – those relevant to the pulse – there is no such precise measurement suggested, even in principle. In fact, very shortly after the passage cited, in which Galen describes the assessment of the speed of a pulse in terms of a knowledge of both the distance covered and time elapsed, he produces a quite different account of the nature of our actual assessment of speed – one which is entirely qualitative in nature.

> We recognise speed and slowness in the first impulse of the artery, but need a great deal of time to discover the relationship between one time and another and one distance and another. So, we do not wait to calculate them for the purpose of the diagnosis of the sick; when we observe something before us, the rush of the impulse is sufficient to indicate its speed; so it is with the artery – one may find that its motion is rushed or relaxed.[41]

A little further on he adds:

---

39 *The Discernment of the Pulse* 3.2 (VIII.889–90 K.)
40 One may compare also a striking passage from the treatise *Mixtures*, where Galen recommends a procedure of comparison of the temperature of bodies at different ages, as discerned by the touch, even suggesting that such a comparison can be carried out in relation to the same body at different ages, with the relevant tactile experiences in some way mentally stored and used much later in the process of such comparison: *Mixtures* 2.9, 52–3 Helmreich (I.590–2 K.). See the commentary ad loc. of Singer and van der Eijk (2018); and further van der Eijk (2015b).
41 *The Discernment of the Pulse* 3.1 (VIII.882 K.).

> The above, then, will be sufficient as indication of the fact that we do not investigate the quantity of the time and distances, but the quality itself of the motion. This is admittedly difficult to express; but if you take what has been said as a basis, and are not completely incapable and useless, you will arrive at the truth without difficulty, in as far as human capacity allows. And even more so, if you practise the discernment of those pulses which are uneven in respect to speed and slowness, you will find that their coming about consists in the quality of the motion. So, for example, in one expansion the starting point of the motion often appears manifestly swifter, but what follows appears slower, and then again the extremity swifter, although we are not measuring certain quantities, whether of times, capacities or distances, but only investigating the quality itself of the motion.[42]

Here, speed is discerned through an immediate perception: quality, quite explicitly, replaces quantity in the mental procedure.

It is noteworthy here that Galen at times explicitly categorizes the variable of 'time' or 'motion' within the pulse under or together with the heading of 'quality', as distinct from 'quantity', which applies to the size of the expansion; see for example the passage cited on p. 142 above (though of course, as we have already seen, 'quantitative' assessment in a modern sense is not applicable to the 'quantity' variable of the pulse, either.)

A couple of other things are worthy of note in these passages. One is the emphasis on 'unevenness' in the latter. What Galen means by this term is an inequality between different *parts* of the pulse. What is apparently stated here, then, is that it is easier, in these qualitative terms, to discern a difference or mismatch between one phase of the motion and another – to make another kind of relative measurement, that is – than to make statements about speed in isolation from such a comparison. Another is a point about the immediate context of these remarks. In the passage immediately preceding the last passage quoted, Galen has given an analysis of perception in terms of primary or minimal perceptible units – an analysis to which we shall turn in a moment – before summing this up with the remark: 'these matters are better philosophized about separately ...' He then turns, as it were, from that 'philosophizing' to the more practical, experiential account of the clinical experience of pulse speed measurement.

The passages just considered may strike us as vague and unsatisfactory. It should, however, be observed that such subjective or immediate perception of speed – again in conjunction with experience, with highly trained senses – is of course all that is available to one in the absence of sophisticated measuring apparatus; that in a number of relevant contexts no such measuring equipment was available until very recent times indeed; and that before its advent professionals in a number of fields to which speed assessment is crucial – sporting

---

[42] *The Discernment of the Pulse* 3.1 (K. VIII.885–6 K.).

and musical, for example, as well as medical – would make such judgements, with a high degree of skill informed by fine-tuned sense training. Indeed, in certain such contexts professional skill and judgement will continue to rely on such assessments, even when quantificatory apparatus is available.

Let us very briefly consider two kinds of example from our contemporary world. First, a modern-day sportsperson – a tennis player, for example, or a cricketer – has always been, and remains, able to make fine judgements of the speed of a particular serve or ground stroke, or of a fast bowler, both in relative terms (X is faster than Y; Z is serving at her fastest today; that was X's slower/faster ball), but also in the terms most relevant to the performance of that sportsperson's skill. That is, such a sportsperson acquires an advanced level of ability to assess which servers, returners or bowlers are fast, medium-paced or indeed exceptionally fast, insofar as those terms relate to that sportsperson's ability at, or difficulty in, playing the balls received. Secondly, in music, any professional – or even reasonably experienced amateur – performer has a highly developed sense not just of relative tempo but of the correct tempo appropriate to a piece of music in a specific genre, as well as an ability to double or halve that tempo, or to perform other subtle transformations of it. There is an internal operation here which has a high degree of accuracy.

In neither case is any technological apparatus – Hawkeye, or a metronome – required to enable the performer to carry out those assessments, or the related motor responses, successfully; where these are available, they will in many cases confirm the accuracy of those judgements.

The same applies, even more strongly – as indeed Galen seems to hint in the passage just considered – to the assessment of the *proportion* or ratio between different time units, that is, to the relative assessment of speeds or time periods which is that involved in the assessment of rhythm. We shall return to this point shortly.

Minimal units of time (1): the atomic nature of time perception

We turn now to a further aspect of Galen's discussion of the assessment of speed – that, indeed, which we saw just now he sums up as a 'philosophizing' on the subject. This is his employment of the notion of minimal – or primarily discernible – units of time.

The conception is to be understood in the context of his attempt to deal with a larger question, which could be summarized as that of the relationship between the raw data of sense perception and our mental processing of them.

For Galen is aware of the problem of the extent to which mental processes or suppositions supply the gaps in the actual content of our perceptual experiences. At one point Galen characterizes the difference as that between things *primarily* and *secondarily* perceived.

> The primary objects of our perception are the experiences within our own bodies; secondary are those which are productive of these, and which underlie them externally. We have a primary perception, in the case of the vehement pulse, of the motion which takes place in the touching parts, as the artery moves away after the pressure; and by virtue of this we state that contraction of the artery is accessible to perception: here, it is accepted that those factors which are productive of the actual experience may be themselves referred to as perceptible.[43]

What Galen is doing, here, is making a point about the fundamental nature of human perception – about how we register, or make sense of, the data available to us in sense perception, and the extent to which this process involves a mental inference from the 'raw data' actually picked up by our sense organs.

The particular relevance of this to the discernment of pulse motion is that one cannot (at least in the above, 'primary' sense) discern the *whole* of the motion of the pulse. The problem is discussed at some length in book 1, chapter 8 of this same text. There is a part of the expansive motion of the pulse which 'eludes perception', both at its beginning and at its end. The motion starts from nothing and at some point becomes strongly perceptible; it seems to be almost a logical consequence of this that there is a time at which the motion has started but is not yet perceptible. One is thus involved in inferential processes, in determining the exact time at which the expansion ends and the first rest starts, and similarly the time at which the first rest stops and the contraction starts. (The problem is even more acute in this latter case, as the contraction is not in any case perceptible in all kinds of pulse – nor, to be sure, as we have seen, by all practitioners.)

There is a part of that motion which is so faint that it escapes actual sense perception, so that we do not, properly speaking, perceive the full extent of the motion and the actual moment at which it comes to an end, but we are able mentally to supply the gap. Similarly, with a motion away from our finger, a loss of pressure: we do not, properly speaking, perceive this motion; nevertheless, through a combination of sense stimuli and inference, the nature of the motion is clear to us.

Galen's use of the concept of minimal units of time, space and motion is connected with this analysis. Our perception of both the passing of time, and the

---

43 *The Discernment of the Pulse* 1.5 (VIII.793 K.).

movement of objects in space, he argues, is an important sense atomistic – there just are minimal units that we actually perceive, in space, time or motion. This is true in spite of the fact that time itself – like the fabric of the universe itself – is *in reality* (*pros phusin*) continuous.

In book 3, chapter 1 of *The Discernment of the Pulse*, Galen talks of 'the impression provided by sense-perception with regard to the discernment of the fast and slow pulses'. He says:

> it is evident [to the senses] that the one readily leaves the places in which it occurs on each occasion and that the other remains there longer, and that the former is, therefore, called swift and the latter is called slow on account of the [nature of the] transitions from places; for sense-perception forms its discernment not in relation to the time of the entire motion, either considered individually and on its own or on the basis of a quantitative comparison. In this respect, our discernment of speed and slowness comes about immediately: it would not come about if we waited to grasp the quantities of the times and distances and then investigate the relations between them, which of course we do not.[44]

That much reads like a prelude to the discussion of the immediate and qualitative nature of our impression of speed which follows a couple of pages later in the text, and which we have already considered. But there is a further, more theoretical, element of the account, which is worth reproducing here in full:

> At the [moment] of the first application of the sense of vision we use some inexpressibly short period of time in order to distinguish the staying in place of the body in motion, and on the basis of that we infer the transition. So, for example, with things that we see from afar, we sometimes have the impression that these remain for a longer time, even if they are moving very fast, and from this it is evident that we distinguish the motion by inference, not by sense-perception. For when any one of the primarily perceptible parts of the body in motion remains in the primarily perceptible place for a primarily perceptible time, then the object seen will seem to be unmoved; but when the primarily perceptible part remains in the primarily perceptible place for a shorter time than that which is primarily perceptible, then it will seem to be in motion. For although in reality each of the things mentioned is capable of being divided *ad infinitum*, in terms of our measuring them by sense-perception they have certain primary and indivisible parts; and from this it is evident that all motion is discerned by inference not by sense-perception. But because of the fact that the inference is closely connected to the sense-perception and the fact that the transition performed by the mind is very fast, it very often seems that the discernment is made not by inference but by sense-perception.
>
> It is only in the case of those things of which the primarily perceptible part remains in the place primary to perception for that time which is primary to perception, that we agree that we are manifestly grasping their motions by inference, not by sense-perception. Examples

---

44 *The Discernment of the Pulse* 3.1 (VIII.883 K.).

are the shadow of a gnomon, the moon, the sun, all the stars and any other things which are most distant from us. But, on the other hand, as stated, when the time is shorter than that which is primary to perception, both the stay and the departure from the places appears to be without duration; for everything which takes place in a time shorter than that which is primary to perception gives the impression of being without duration.[45]

Both space and time are, for Galen, infinitely subdivisible. Our perception, however, takes place on the basis of minimal units of each, below which it does not go. What is happening in our actual perceptual apparatus, at the most granular level, in our perception of motion, is that we discern an object at point X1 and then discern it having ceased to be at point X1 and appearing at point X2. We do not *actually* discern it in motion: the motion is something that we infer on the basis of its disappearance from X1 and appearance at X2. And an analogous procedure applies to our perception of the passage of time. What Galen is saying might be elucidated by an anachronistic example, that of frames in a film. Even though any motion, and the time in which that motion happens, are *in their nature* continuous, not atomistic, our own perception of both the motion and time is best understood in terms of frames – units than which we cannot perceive anything smaller. Our perception of motion, and therefore of speed, comes about through our registering of the quick succession of these frames.

Of course, most of the time we do not realize that this is what is happening – that our minds are in some sense supplying the impression of motion, whereas all we see are frames. This is why Galen introduces the examples of distant, or of very slow-moving, objects, to illustrate the principle. Here – for example in the progress of a shadow around a sundial – we may stare as long as we like, but we will not *perceive* a motion; we will, however, after some time see that the shadow has moved from one place to another. Here, then, we infer that there has been motion; and in this case we are conscious of the fact that we are making an inference. In normal cases of motion perception, Galen is saying, we are also making such inferences as part of the perceptive process, but this is happening at a subconscious level.

So, Galen's concept of minimal units of space and time belongs within his account of the fundamental nature of sense-perception, and relates to phenomena which take place at the most microscopic level, as it were at the edge of our consciousness of the perception. It is part of his account of the relationship between the role of the sense organs and mental inputs in our sense-making.[46]

---

45 *The Discernment of the Pulse* 3.1 (VIII.883–5 K.).
46 These issues are further explored in Singer (2022).

As a coda to this theoretical discussion of minimal time units in Galen, and its relationship to his view of time as in its nature continuous, it is interesting to consider the later arguments of the Platonist philosopher Damascius. Damascius seems to have combined an account of time 'leaping', rather than moving continuously, with the view that such leaps are divisible, and in fact infinitely so. The combination of ideas is challenging, and detailed interpretation beyond our scope here. It seems, however, that he argued that time was *in its nature* divided into parts, but *conceptually* infinitely divisible – thus in a sense reversing the Galenic picture of a continuum in nature which our human perception translates into an atomic structure. Damascius is here addressing the problem of the relationship of the 'now' to the flow of time, with the related paradox – a feature of the debate from Aristotle onward – of the ceasing instant, or of how the present turns into the past.[47] His discussion is thus fundamentally conceptual in nature, whereas Galen's is fundamentally concerned with the nature of our perception; but the parallel, and indeed reversal, provide a point of curiosity, at the very least.

Minimal units of time (2): the analysis of rhythm

The notion of minimal or 'primary' time units arises also in a different context, however, which is also worthy of our attention: that of the analysis of rhythm.

Both Galen and his predecessor in pulse theory, Herophilus of Chalcedon, were concerned to measure the rhythm of a pulse. Although there are differences of detail, essentially the rhythm of a pulse is understood as ratio, namely that between the time taken by the expansion and the time taken by the contrac-

---

47 Damascius states that 'time always flows, and progresses by leaps (*halmata*), in accordance with the nature of a progression by intervals', that 'these leaps are measures of time, defined by demiurgic divisions (*dēmiourgikais tomais*)' and that the now 'is so called not as a limit of time but as time which is demiurgically indivisible (*ameriston*), even if it is divisible in our conception – and that infinitely', *Doubts and Solutions on Plato's Parmenides*, III.191–2 Westerink and Combès (II.241–2 Ruelle). For discussion see Sorabji 1983: 55–6. Combès understands the expression 'demiurgic divisions' (that is, divisions due to the creator or original creation of the cosmos), which occurs also in Damascius' *Doubts and Solutions on First Principles* (II.178 Westerink and Combès, I.198 Ruelle), as derived from Plato's account of the construction, and divisions, of the world soul at *Timaeus* 35b4–36d7; in any case the sense must be of a division which is intrinsic to the object, as distinct from what is brought to it by our conception. The context of this passage is a commentary on the discussion of the relationship of the One to time in Plato's *Parmenides*, and within this Platonist framework Damascius is also exercised to give an account of time which in some way combines being and indivisibility with coming-to-be and motion.

tion.⁴⁸ Herophilus in fact seems to have paid particular attention to this feature of the pulse, and Galen follows him in this, while criticizing him in detail.⁴⁹

In a way which recalls our discussion in chapter 2 of the medical understanding of four main phases of life, Herophilus identified a normal pulse rhythm, as well as a normal pulse speed, and a normal pulse frequency, for each of these four ages.

Within those, we shall focus here especially on the question of the assessment of *rhythm*, while that of *puknotēs* (which we already encountered) will receive its own discussion below. But a little should be said about the assessment of *speed*, too, as the interpretation of Herophilus' theory here is of relevance to a broader question of the nature of the standard or objective basis of measurement which is a recurrent problem for us in this chapter.

For the question arises here, what level of normalization is in play. In stating that there is a speed, frequency or rhythm of pulse that is normal for children, is Herophilus referring to a norm that should be taken as applying universally, to all children of a certain age, or is he rather at pains to identify the normal speed (etc.) *for each individual child?* The parallel with the discussion of *puknotēs*, where it seems clear that Herophilus does indeed posit a norm – and in this case, an objectively measurable one – of universal applicability to *all* individuals of a certain age, in conjunction with the arguments of Berrey, suggests that we should favour the former interpretation.⁵⁰ If that is correct, then it seems that, at least *theoretically*, that speed might be expressible as a definite quantity, and not only in terms of the observer's impression; and the discussion of frequency below suggests that Herophilus might in principle have had the ambition to provide such objective measurements. If this is right, then even though there would seem to be strong limitations on the feasibility of such measurements in the ancient context, the ambition of Herophilus to perform them would constitute a significant difference between him and Galen – and doubtless part of the background to Galen's attack on him for excessive claims to precision, which we shall come to shortly.

---

48 According to the more precise analysis mentioned above (pp. 138–9), the ratio in question is in fact that of the whole time taken by the expansion plus the former rest period (E + R1) to the whole time taken by the contraction plus the latter rest period (C + R2). It seems that Herophilus' account does not include mention of the periods of rest; at least, Galen repeatedly accuses him of confusion or unclarity as to whether it is included or not (see especially *The Discernment of the Pulse* 3.3, VIII.911–12 K.).
49 For detailed interpretation of Herophilus' views in this area see Berrey (2017); fundamental for the text and interpretation of the testimonia to Herophilus is von Staden (1989).
50 Berrey (2017): 200–1.

Let us turn to Herophilus' account of the differential pulse *rhythms* to be found at different ages. Summarizing and combining the evidence from two main testimonia, we may paint the following picture: Herophilus connected each stage of a life with a different rhythm, and in doing so drew closely and explicitly on the terminology of musical and metrical theory. Each phase of life corresponds to one of the four rhythms, pyrrhic (˘ ˘), trochee (¯ ˘), spondee (¯ ¯), iambus (˘ ¯), where the first beat in each case corresponds to the expansion of the pulse, and the second to its contraction. Secondly, he equated the expansion with the metrical or musical term *arsis* ('upbeat') and the contraction with the *thesis* ('downbeat'). Thirdly, again following metrical theory, he understood the units underlying these rhythms in terms of 'primary time units': a metrical short syllable corresponds to one unit, a long syllable to two.[51] Thus, the pulse in the newborn consists of two units, that of the youth and the post-prime or old person to three units, that of the prime to four units.

In spite of his own adoption of the theory of primary perceptible time units in a different context, already noted, Galen has considerable criticisms of Herophilus' theory here. One point of departure seems to be that although Galen does discuss the importance of the relationship between the two main parts of the pulse, Herophilus gives this notion of rhythm much more prominence and technical importance in his system. Though complete clarity about Herophilus' system, and therefore about the nature of Galen's criticisms of it, is impossible, it seems too that Herophilus claims both a level of precision, and a universalizability, for his time units, which Galen rejects.

Part of Galen's criticism is undoubtedly based on his view, already discussed, that it is impossible precisely to discern the pulse throughout its entire duration: a part of it eludes perception. This throws doubt on Herophilus' project of providing precise mathematical proportions for each pulse. Moreover, he takes Herophilus to be unclear and probably inconsistent about the parts of the pulse: is he taking into account the periods of rest, or not (see note 48 above)?

---

[51] The two passages are Rufus, *Synopsis on the Pulse* 4, 223–5 Daremberg and Ruelle (von Staden 1989, no. 177 and Galen, *Synopsis on the Pulse* 12, IX.463–5 Kühn (von Staden 1989, no. 183). There are some difficulties in detail of interpretation (especially the characterization of the newborn's pulse as *alogos*, 'without ratio', attributed to Herophilus in the former text), as well as differences in detail (for example the mention of *arsis* and *thesis* appears in the latter text but not the former; the latter attributes to Herophilus the terminology, already encountered above, of 'primary perceptible time units', whereas the former says only 'primary time units'). Part of Herophilus' claim here, at least on the basis of the second text, seems to be that the primary time unit is itself established on basis of observation of the newborn child.

The latter point – Herophilus' unclarity on parts of the pulse – certainly forms part of Galen's criticism at the end of the second of our main testimonies. Here he states that Herophilus' equation of the newborn's pulse with two equal time units is consistent with his measuring the contraction from its beginning, whereas in his claim that the contraction of the pulse in old people can extend as far as ten primary time units, he must be counting the contraction from the end of the expansion, that is including the whole period of the rest as part of the contraction.

The former point, meanwhile – the impossibility of discerning the duration of the pulse in its entirety – seems to underlie his criticism of the Herophilean account in another passage:

> Why, then, did Herophilus assume some primary perceptible time by measurement against which he says that the other times are two, three or more in length, either in terms of units which are complete and, as they themselves call them, 'non-lengthened', or in units which are slightly, considerably or very much increased? For he seems to write this as though he were discerning the times in the cases of all the pulses precisely, either the times of the motions alone or also of those of the periods of rest after those times (for this makes no difference in relation to our present difficulty) ...[52]

Both from this passage itself and from its preceding context it is clear that part of Galen's issue is with Herophilus' implicit claim to be able to measure the time lengths precisely, as a basis for the establishment of the 'rhythms'. To put it simply: Herophilus cannot perform the measurements in the way required by his system. There is, perhaps, a further criticism too, of the Herophilean ambition to produce precise mathematical proportion. That is: even if Herophilus *could* produce the precise measurements in the way that would be needed, he would be wrong to believe that what will result is a series of neat mathematical ratios. This (Galen would be arguing) is an inappropriate attempt to impose a mathematical or musical system on the observed reality. The clinical reality is messier and more nuanced.

This latter interpretation of Galen's criticism is perhaps supported by the following passage, from another of Galen's pulse treatises, where – this time without reference to Herophilus – he outlines the notion of the rhythmic relationship of the expansion and the contraction, again making reference to mathematical proportion:

> This [*sc. the inequality of the expansion and the contraction*] arises sometimes in virtue of an expressible difference, sometimes in virtue of an inexpressible one. There are two ways in

---

[52] *The Discernment of the Pulse* 3.3 (VIII.913 K.).

which it may be expressible, either as a multiple, or as a ratio between numbers, [of the sort] known also as an epimoric ratio.[53] Multiples are: double, triple, quadruple, and so on. Ratios between numbers [arise] where to an expansion which lasts two units of time there corresponds a contraction which lasts five, seven, nine or eleven. There is then a threefold distinction within the whole [category] of the inexpressibles overall: for either the time of the expansion is inexpressible, or that of the contraction, or both. Each of these individually sometimes has the inexpressible times augmented slightly – whether there is a plurality of these, or whether there is one primary one – and sometimes to a greater extent and sometimes to the greatest extent. And of course, 'primary time' should not be understood in terms of its actual nature, but with respect to our sense-perception. For this is how it is with musicians too. ...[54]

There is a certain amount that is not perfectly clear here, and up to a point at least Galen could here be taken to be summarizing the system elsewhere attributed to Herophilus. But he mentions a range of possible proportions beyond those explicitly attributed to Herophilus; and the 'inexpressibility' mentioned seems best taken in the mathematical sense, whereby an 'inexpressible' difference is one which cannot be reduced to a ratio between integers. The alternative would be to take 'inexpressible' here as simply meaning 'unquantifiable' or 'uncertain in extent'. On either interpretation, Galen is again expressing himself sceptically in relation to the neat simplicity which is the ambition of the Herophilean. The latter represents a distortion of the full range of empirical realities.

Before concluding this section it will be helpful to return the theoretical account of Aristoxenus, and investigate in more detail his account of the role of the minima, or 'primary time units'. This seems to constitute an important part of the theoretical background to the discussions that we have been considering; and the points of contact as well as departure will be instructive.

> Time is divided by 'rhythmizables', within each of its parts. There are three such 'rhythmizables': speech (*lexis*), song (*melos*) and bodily motion. A 'primary time unit' (*prōtos chronos*) is one which cannot be divided by any of the rhythmizables.[55]

---

53 The usual context of this terminology was Greek music theory, where an epimoric ration is typically understood as one which takes the form n:n+1 (see Barker 1994: 117); in more general terms, it is defined as a ratio between numbers where the larger one contains both the smaller one and a simple fraction of it; cf. John Philoponus, *On Aristotle's Posterior Analytics* 13.3, 160, giving as examples the ratios 2:3 (3 is the sum of 2 and one-half of 2) and 3:5 (5 is the sum of 3 and two-thirds of three). Galen's usage seems consistent with this, provided that we include improper fractions (e.g. 7 is the sum of 2 and five-halves of 2).
54 *The Distinct Types of Pulse* 1.8 (VIII.516–17 K.).
55 Aristoxenus, *Elements of Rhythm* 2.9–11, 6–8 Pearson.

Here it seems clear that a *prōtos chronos* is to be understood as context-dependent: it is a unit established in each case in accordance with a particular kind of motion, musical performance or speech act. We are not here talking about a standard or unit with any kind of universal applicability; the standard is set and established within a particular performative context, then used as a basis for further measurement and assessment within that context. A letter is the minimum unit of speech, as a particular motion, for example in a dance, is the minimum unit of bodily motion, and the primary time unit is that taken for the performance or utterance of any such minimal unit. The actual time span corresponding to the primary unit will, however, vary from case to case. But whatever the length of that established primary unit, all further patterns of time, and in particular rhythms, within the performance or utterance will be based on that unit.

Aristoxenus' discussion could be interpreted as relevant to both Galen's account of the physiological limits of human perception – there simply are units below which we cannot perceive – and of the Herophilean one, which is concerned rather with the construction or recognition of rhythms, for example by a musician or a doctor, on the basis of acknowledged and recognized minimal units established in a particular context. It is the latter analysis which is relevant to the discussion of rhythm. Neither Aristoxenus in his description of a minimal time unit in the sense relevant to the establishment of rhythm, nor Herophilus in his use of this conception in this context, need be concerned with a universal human constant. It is within the individual musical performance, or – in the context relevant to medical diagnosis – the individual bodily motion, that the norm, that is, the relevant 'minimal unit' is established, as a kind of analytical building block.

The assessment of rhythms is conducted in purely relative terms (whether or not that is the case for the assessment of speed and of frequency, as already discussed). All that is at stake with the measurement of rhythm is that we can make a mental assessment of two time periods and on that basis establish the ratio between them. Of course, the question still arises as to how, mentally, the assessment of time units that go to make up the rhythm in question is performed. Again, however – as in the discussion of the 'immediate' or qualitative assessment of speed, above – that is a question that arises today as much as in the ancient world. Such assessment of the relationship between two (or more) time units is an absolutely standard feature of music-making and indeed music perception. The mathematical relationship between two short time lengths can be, and regularly is, assessed to a high degree of accuracy, without the involvement of any independent measuring device – or even any objective metric – to measure the length of the time units involved.

Summary on minimal time units in Aristoxenus, Herophilus and Galen

On the basis of the above, it seems that Galen's 'primary perceptible times' perform a significantly different role from those of Aristoxenus. Galen's main use of the conception is in the context of his account of the nature of our interconnected perception of time, motion and speed, where his central claim is that there are, from the perceptual point of view, minimal units of both time and space, and that our perception of motion and speed arises from the succession of these.

'Primary times' in Aristoxenus are, to the contrary, units chosen arbitrarily, or in certain contexts, on the basis of which other time units, in particular rhythms, are constructed. They are in no sense constants of, or in themselves intrinsic to, human perception. (Galen's use of the term in the last passage cited from him, pp. 155–6 above, may perhaps be taken in this sense rather than in that observed in his account of the perception of motion.)

In Herophilus, meanwhile, though the situation is less clear, it seems that 'primary times' are, at least in some contexts, taken as universals not just of human perception but of human physiology: they are (perhaps) universals, and correspond to the smallest duration observed in the phases of the pulse, in childhood and then in subsequent ages. They can also be taken as fundamental – in a way that Aristoxenus or Galen might also accept – in the construction of rhythm, but Herophilus apparently accords them a universalizing status, as well as a level of precision in the way they can be employed, which Galen certainly rejects.

In conclusion, I suggest that our analysis so far has pointed to a rather close parallel between Aristoxenus and Galen in their scientific procedure, in particular in the way in which they both use mathematical models.

It is noteworthy that both Aristoxenus and Galen are continuum theorists: for them atomic units, or minima, are pragmatic constructs which help to explain certain aspects of reality, or how we measure it. Aristoxenus' 'primary times' are not, any more than Galen's, intrinsic features of the physical reality. Rather, they are of pragmatic use – indeed absolutely necessary – for us, as practising musicians. They are intellective or conceptual tools by which we divide, and make sense of, time.[56]

---

56 Aristoxenus' combination of continuous with non-continuous concepts is perhaps still clearer in his theory of pitch intervals, which provides an instructive parallel, even if it takes us some way from notions relevant to time. Here, departing from the Pythagorean tradition which was only concerned with intervals understood in terms of precise points, given by mathematical proportions, Aristoxenus states that the number of pitches available between any two other pitches

A broader intellectual or strategic similarity between the two authors may be suggested. Both are fundamentally concerned, not with theoretical or mathematical entities, but with observable and practical realities – musical on the one hand, medical on the other. For both, the mathematical model or calculation, to the extent that one is used, is a heuristic tool to enable the practitioner to carry out observations, or performances, in a way appropriate to the underlying reality, which is *not* itself an abstract mathematical object. In this context, Aristoxenus departed from a whole tradition, the Pythagorean, which took numbers and mathematical models to be the prior entities, insisting rather on the priority of the heard reality, in relation to which the mathematical model offers a tool of some, but limited, usefulness and validity.[57] Galen departs from the apparently Herophilean insistence on the mathematical model as something which offers a precise correspondence to the reality of rhythms manifested by the human body; for him such a model can be at best an approximation, and its use is subordinate to the informed fine training of the senses.

An isolated case of quantification? Pulse rate and the water-clock

In all the above the question has arisen of the benchmark or standard against which any measurement of time units, or of speed, might be made; and we have repeatedly found ourselves in a conceptual world in which there is no absolute or independent standard of measurement, let alone measuring apparatus.

And yet there is one apparent exception to this for which we have evidence in the ancient sources.

---

is potentially infinite. The view has strong practical and aesthetic consequences. It is not just that the *lichanos*, for example (roughly equivalent to our 'third'), can be pitched at several distinct points over the range of a whole tone, in accordance with the different 'kinds' (*genē*, roughly 'scales'). It is that that range is, in theory, infinitely subdivisible: there is theoretically an infinite number of thirds (νοητέον ... ἀπείρους τὸν ἀριθμὸν τὰς λιχάνους) (*Elements of Harmonics* 1.26). All notes within such a range will be heard as, and should be defined as, thirds, though they will all be subtly different thirds. He also, however, identifies a unit arrived at by precise mathematical division, namely that of a twelfth of a tone, which may be used to provide a mathematical solution to the problem of the consistent calculation of intervals (1.25). This precise mathematical division does not correspond to any 'real' musical entity, and in a sense divides the musical spectrum in an arbitrary manner; but the minimal units thus arrived at are again of practical use to the musician in the calibration of larger intervals.

57 For analysis of Aristoxenus along these lines see Barker (1978), (2005); Litchfield (1988).

In the context of an account by a later medical author, Marcellinus, of his approach to fever, Herophilus is said to have identified excessive size, vehemence and frequency (*puknotēs*)[58] as key diagnostic signs. Frequency, indeed, takes on a particular prominence in another testimony for the theory and practice of Herophilus:

> Frequency of the pulse is first established[59] when the fever starts and remains until the final dissolution. A story goes that Herophilus placed such confidence in 'pulse frequency', using it as a sure sign, that he constructed a *clepsydra* containing a precise amount [of water], specified according to the normal pulse at each age; he would arrive at the patient's bedside, set up the *clepsydra* and feel the pulse of the person with fever; he would declare that the pulse was 'more frequent', that is that the patient had more (or less) fever, in accordance with the amount by which the motions of the pulse exceeded the normal number, in relation to the filling of the *clepsydra*.[60]

Although there are other possibilities, it seems most likely that the type of water-clock attributed to Herophilus here at the patient's bedside is one involving inflow to a marked vessel, the various markings corresponding to the time taken for a certain number of pulse beats to be completed by a 'normal' patient, of various ages.

So, what is the significance of what Herophilus (according to Marcellinus) is doing here? One obvious answer is that he is showing off – presenting himself at the patient's bedside with a tool which asserts his superior knowledge and accuracy in relation to that of his rivals, and thus commands confidence.

In more technical, or internal terms, what he is doing is measuring the *puknotēs* of the pulse. We have already considered in some detail Galen's treatment of this concept, and the difficulty of equating it straightforwardly with 'pulse rate'. Before proceeding we should pause to consider whether Herophilus' conception is the same as Galen's, or whether there may be a significant difference. Marcellinus, the author who gives us this piece of evidence, in fact also gives us, a little earlier in the same text, an explicit definition of *puknotēs* and of the distinction between it and speed (*tachutēs*).[61] The account he gives seems to be a

---

[58] For the problem of translation of this term see above, pp. 137–8, with n. 29; in spite of the reservation made there, I use 'frequency' in this present context in the interest of readability.
[59] Berrey translates: 'frequency becomes primary'; it seems to me rather that the word *puknotēs* is here being used to refer to 'increased frequency' (just as, by a similar semantic stretch, commented on by Galen, *megethos* can mean both 'size' in the abstract sense of 'magnitude' and also 'bigness').
[60] Marcellinus, *The Pulse* 11, 463 Schöne (= no. 182 in von Staden 1989).
[61] Marcellinus, *The Pulse* 6, 460–1 Schöne. Unfortunately, the date of Marcellinus, as well as his relationship to either Herophilus or Galen, is unclear. Clearly, he is writing some time after Her-

common-sense one. You are said to go to the country quickly if you complete the journey there quickly, whereas you are said to go there *puknōs* if the interval of days between your journeys is a short one. This seems potentially to bypass the complexity and subtlety we saw above in Galen's account, whereby he was enabled to treat *puknotēs* as something discernible within one beat. If so – that is, if *puknotēs* is defined by Herophilus simply as the 'frequency', as the shortness or length of time between one beat and the next – then the way is indeed open for him to measure it, in a way that it is not for Galen – and indeed, in a way recognizable to us as 'pulse rate'.

And indeed, some such measurement, in a form not dissimilar to its modern descendants, seems to be what is attributed to Herophilus in the above text. We note the distinctive features of *puknotēs* (in that 'common-sense' understanding, as just specified) that make it accessible to this form of measurement. In the problematic case of speed, considered above, we had a distance travelled and a space of time which would elude any ancient measuring technology. Speed, as understood by both Herophilus and Galen, could admit of no such technology-based measurement. Here, by contrast, we have a clearly countable number – that of the beats – and a time period which is long enough to be measurable by a standard, though carefully calibrated, water-clock. By focussing on frequency – in our terms, 'rate' – rather than speed, then, and thus on two clearly quantifiable figures – number of beats and a longer, and thus measurable, time span – one is, at least in this narrow context, replacing the finely trained human apparatus of tactile assessment and observation with an independent standard. One is, in fact, 'measuring the pulse' according to exactly the same principle by which it was later measured – and sometimes still is – in the modern period, with the advent of portable watches.

How much significance or influence such a quantificatory approach had, even within the narrow context of the 'frequency' of the pulse (which, as we have seen, was to ancient practitioners but one amongst many variables), is unanswerable, certainly on the basis of this isolated ancient report. If the report is to be relied upon, then we seem to have yet another instance of the methodological gulf between Herophilus in Galen, in relation to measurement and quantification, Herophilus here claiming to offer precise measurement of a sort which Galen would never suggest – and which, indeed, as we have seen, is in principle impossible, given Galen's definition of *puknotēs*.

---

ophilus; and some have taken the fact that he does not mention Galen as indicating that he predates the latter. On the other hand, some of the terminology and language he uses seems quite close to Galen's.

Whatever the currency of the quantificatory method attributed to Herophilus in this account, however, it was undoubtedly the model of the individual practitioner's highly trained senses and expert skills of analysis that remained by far the dominant one – as, indeed, it had to, in a world where so small a part of the observable phenomena taken to be relevant to medicine could admit of any kind of quantification or precise measurement. (See figure 15.)

It should be mentioned, however, as a coda, that the musical or metrical model of pulse assessment enjoyed great influence in later times, constituting one aspect of ancient pulse theory that was taken up with particular enthusiasm, especially in the Renaissance.[62]

Conclusion

A number of fundamental conceptual or philosophical points, then, emerge from Galen's and other technical discussions of time in relation to motion, alongside several points of practical or clinical significance.

The conceptual or philosophical points may be summarized as follows:

(1) Our perception of time is – according to Galen, but in contradiction of the Aristotelian tradition – *sui generis:* neither the abstract conception of time nor our human perception of depends on that of motion.
(2) Our perception of speed – though its precise quantification or measurement is possible in theory, and on the larger scale also in practice – is, again according to Galen, fundamentally qualitative at the 'micro' level, and therefore is so in many clinical contexts.
(3) Although time, like space, is continuous in its structure, it may be usefully divided into minimal or atomic units, especially in the context of the establishment of ratios or rhythms. According to Galen, our perception of the passing of time, as of the motion of objects – and therefore also of speed – takes place on the basis of such minimal units, that is, time is atomic in its structure from the point of view of perception, even though in its true nature it is not. According to other theorists, such minimal or atomic time units may either (a) correspond to universal physiological realities, or (b) represent divisions of the time continuum which are of crucial pragmatic value, although they are not there 'in nature'.

---

62 See e.g. Siraisi (1975).

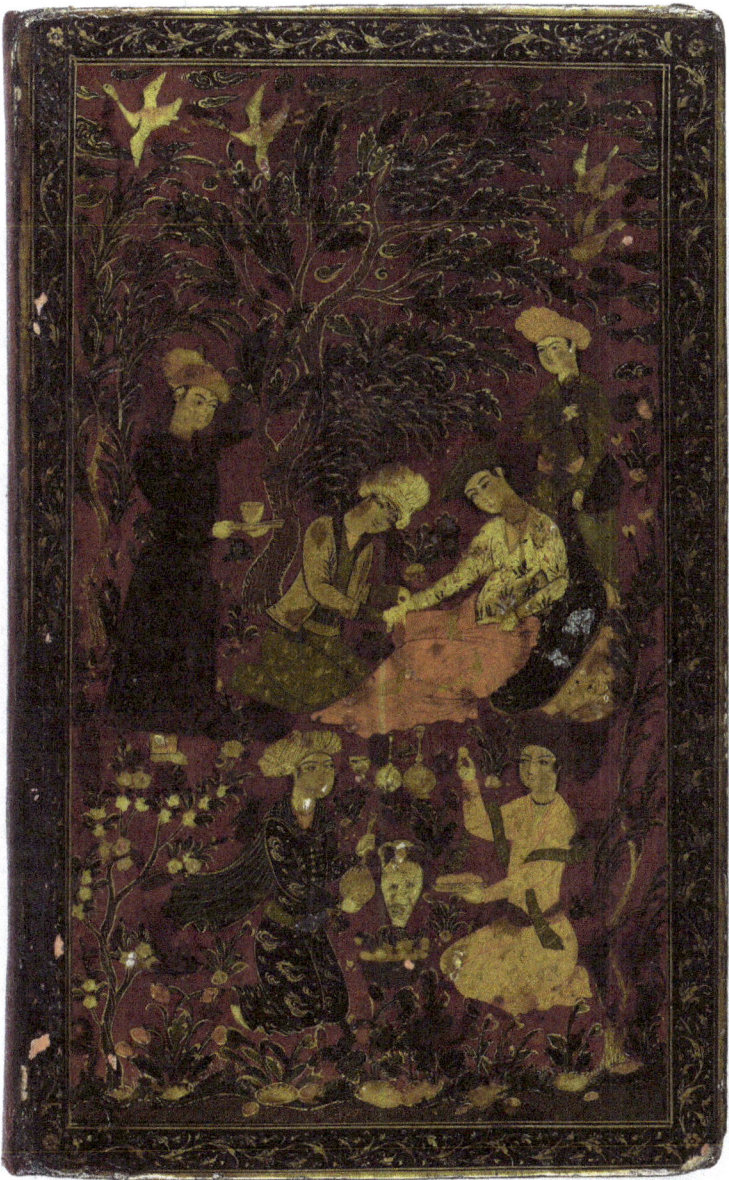

Figure 15: The fine-tuning of the senses (2): the hands and the pulse. A doctor takes a woman's pulse. From a manuscript of Avicenna's Canon, image from Wellcome Collection, London

More important, though, than these theoretical analyses and considerations, in practical terms – and more important for Galen and Aristoxenus – is the notion that it is possible to develop and fine-tune our senses in a way relevant to clinical (or musical) practice, the notion of a rationally informed training and technical expertise arising in response to the challenges of time, speed and rhythm. Of course, there is little in Galen's theoretical medical model, in his diagnostic judgements or therapeutic recommendations – or in those of his predecessors, such as Herophilus – that we would find persuasive. We will not be concerned to measure or assess the same variables that they claimed to, nor will we find their specific claims for their success in measurement or assessment of them convincing. In Galen's assertion of the notions of fine-tuned sense training, however, and of its complex relationship with verbal reasoning and mental conceptions on the one hand, and radical experiential incommunicability, on the other, as well as in his statement of their potential relevance to the practice of an art, he makes a unique contribution to ancient technical, medical and philosophical thought, and one which presents points of interest and challenge for us today.

Our study has revealed the fundamental significance of time awareness, time assessment and time management in the ancient world, in a variety of experiential and scientific contexts. The particular ways in which this significance manifests itself, in terms of medical and philosophical theories, social and cultural preoccupations, and measuring technologies, are strikingly different in the Graeco-Roman world from their instantiation in the globalized twenty-first century. Different, too, in particular, is the balance between the competing claims of quantification and precision and those of educated sense training and subjective judgement. We have, however, seen anxieties, concerns and intellectual ambitions which are in many ways familiar, playing themselves out in a very unfamiliar – and constantly surprising – historical theatre.

Bibliography

Primary Texts

Citation conventions and abbreviations
Where a text has cited by a particular modern edition, the details of that edition are given here; otherwise I have simply listed the authors and texts cited (using standard English translations of their titles). Texts of 'Hippocrates' and Galen have been cited by page number in the standard nineteenth-century editions of Littré (L.) and Kühn (K.) respectively; in some cases they have also been cited by page number of a more recent edition, usually that of either CMG or Loeb (see below).

Where a text has been cited according to page numbers of a CAG, CMG or Loeb edition, then that edition is listed below simply by editor, series volume number, and date; in other cases of modern editions, the full bibliographical details are given.

CAG Commenatria in Aristotelem Graeca, 23 volumes, Berlin: Reimer, 1882–1909, repr. Berlin: de Gruyter.
CMG Corpus Medicorum Graecorum, Lepizig: Teubner: Berlin: Akademie-Verlag and Berlin: de Gruyter, 1914–.
     Texts freely available on line, most with parallel English or other modern translation, at: http://cmg.bbaw.de/epubl/online/editionen.html
DK   H. Diels and W. Kranz, *Fragmente der Vorsokratiker*, 6th edition, Berlin: Weidmann, 1952.
K.   C. G. Kühn, *Galeni Opera Omnia*, 22 volumes, Leipzig, 1821–33, repr. Hildesheim: Olms, 1964–5.
     Texts freely available on line at: https://www.biusante.parisdescartes.fr/histoire/medica/resultats/index.php?tout=galien%20kühn&op=OU&statut=charge&fille=o&cotemere=45674
L.   E. Littré, *Oeuvres complètes d' Hippocrate*, 10 volumes, Paris, 1839–61
     Texts freely available on line at: https://www.biusante.parisdescartes.fr/histoire/medica/resultats/index.php?fille=o&cotemere=34859
Loeb Loeb Classical Library, Cambridge, MA: Harvard University Press, 1912– .
     Texts available on line (with subscription), at: https://www.loebclassics.com.
SVF J. von Arnim, *Stoicorum Veterum Fragmenta*, 3 volumes, Leipzig: Teubner, 1903–5, repr. 1964.

List of primary sources cited

Aeneas Tacticus

Aeschines
The False Embassy

Aëtius of Amida
Medical Books

Anthologia Palatina

Aristotle
Historia Animalium
Physics
Poetics
Politics
Respiration
Rhetoric

ps.-Aristotle
The Athenian Constitution

Aristoxenus
Elements of Harmonics, ed. H. Macran, *The Harmonics of Aristoxenus*, Oxford: Clarendon Press, reprinted Hildesheim: Olms, 1974.
Elements of Rhythm, ed. L. Pearson, *Aristoxenus: Elementa Rhythmica*, Oxford: Clarendon Press, 1990.

Arrian
Discourses of Epictetus

Athenaeus
The Dinner Sophists

Augustine
The City of God
Confessions

Caesar
Gallic War

Cicero
Letters to Friends
On the Orator
The Orator
Tusculan Disputations

Damascius
Doubts and Solutions on Plato's Parmenides, ed., commentary and trans. L. G. Westerink and J. Combès, *Damascius: Commentaire du Parménide de Platon*, vol. III, Paris: Les Belles Lettres, 2002; ed. C. A. Ruelle, *Damascius Diadochus Dubitationes et Solutiones in Platonis Parmenidem*, vol. II, Paris, 1889, repr. Amsterdam: Hakkert, 1966.

Demosthenes
Against Euboulides
Against Konon
Against Makartatos
Against Stephanos
On the Crown

Dio Cassius

Diogenes Laertius
Lives of the Eminent Philosophers

Galen
Affections and Errors of the Soul, ed. W. de Boer, CMG V 4,1,1, 1937, English translation in Singer (2013).
Anatomical Procedures, those parts of the text which survive only in Arabic translated by M. Simon, *Sieben Bücher Anatomie des Galen*, II, Leipzig: Hinrich'sche Buchhandlung, 1906.
Bloodletting against Erasistratus
Commentary on Hippocrates' Aphorisms
Commentary on Hippocrates' Epidemics, book 1, ed. E. Wenkebach and F. Pfaff, CMG V 10,1, 1934.
Commentary on Hippocrates' Epidemics, book 6, ed. E. Wenkebach and F. Pfaff, CMG V 10,2,2, 1956.
Commentary on Hippocrates' The Nature of the Human Being, ed. J. Mewaldt, CMG V 9,1, 1914.
Crises, ed. B. Alexanderson, *Galenos Περὶ κρίσεων, Überlieferung und Text*, Studia Graeca et Latina Gothoburgensia 23, Göteborg: Elanders Boktryckeri Arktiebolag.
Critical Days
The Discernment of the Pulse
The Distinct Types of Fever
The Distinct Types of Pulse
The Doctrines of Hippocrates and Plato, ed. with English translation P. De Lacy, CMG V 4,1,2, 3 volumes, 1978–84, new edition 2005.
An Exhortation to Study the Arts, ed. A. Barigazzi, CMG V 1,1, 1991, English translation in Singer (1997).
Health (De sanitate tuenda), ed. K. Koch, CMG V 4,2, 1923, English translation in Singer (forthcoming).
Mixtures, ed. G. Helmreich, *Galeni De temperamentis libri tres*, Leipzig: Teubner, 1904, English translation in Singer and van der Eijk (2018).

The Order of My Own Books, ed. I. Müller, in *Claudii Galeni Pergameni Scripta Minora*, vol. II, Leipzig: Teubner 1891, also ed. with French translation in V. Boudon-Millot, *Galien: Oeuvres, Tome I*, Paris: Les Belles Lettres, English translation in Singer (1997).
My Own Books, ed. I. Müller, in *Claudii Galeni Pergameni Scripta Minora*, vol. II, Leipzig: Teubner 1891, also ed. with French translation in V. Boudon-Millot, *Galien: Oeuvres, Tome I*, Paris: Les Belles Lettres, English translation in Singer (1997).
Periods (*Adversus eos qui de typis scripserunt, vel de circuitibus*)
The Pulse for Beginners, English translation in Singer (1997)
Prognosis, ed. V. Nutton, CMG V 8,1, 1979.
The Shaping of the Embryo, ed. D. Nickel, CMG V 3,3, 2001, English translation in Singer (1997).
The Soul's Dependence on the Body, ed. I. Müller, in *Claudii Galeni Pergameni Scripta Minora*, vol. II, Leipzig: Teubner, 1891, English translation in Singer (2013).
Synopsis on the Pulse
The Therapeutic Method
The Therapeutic Method to Glaucon

Aulus Gellius
Attic Nights

Euripides
Hippolytus

Herodotus
Histories

Hesiod
Works and Days

'Hippocrates'
Affections, ed. and trans. P. Potter, Loeb V, 1988.
Airs, Waters, Places, ed. H. Diller, CMG I 1,2, 1970, new edition 2002.
Aphorisms, ed. and trans. W. H. S. Jones, Loeb IV, 1931.
Diseases 1–2, ed. and trans. P. Potter, Loeb V, 1988.
Diseases 3, ed. and trans. P. Potter, Loeb VI, 1988.
Diseases 4, ed. and trans. P. Potter, Loeb X, 2012.
Diseases of Girls ed. and trans. P. Potter, Loeb IX, 2010.
Epidemics, books 1 and 3, ed. and trans. W. H. S. Jones, Loeb I, 1923.
Epidemics, books 2 and 4–7, ed. and trans. W. D. Smith, Loeb VII, 1994
Hebdomads
Internal Affections, ed. and trans. P. Potter, Loeb VI, 1988.
The Nature of the Human Being, ed. J. Jouanna, CMG I 1,3, 1975, new edition 2002.
Prognostic, ed. and trans. W. H. S. Jones, Loeb II, 1923.
Regimen, ed. R. Joly and S. Byl, CMG I 2,4, new edition 2003.
Regimen in Acute Diseases, ed. and trans. W. H. S. Jones, Loeb II, 1923.
Regimen in Health, see *The Nature of the Human Being*

Homer
Odyssey

Horace
The Art of Poetry

Marcellinus
The Pulse, ed. H. Schöne, 'Markellinos' Pulslehre: ein griechsiches Anekdoton', in *Festschrift zur 49. Versammlung deutscher Philologen und Schulmänner*, 448–72, Basel: Birkhauser, 1907.

Marcus Aurelius
Meditations

Ovid
Metamorphoses

Petronius
Satyricon

John Philoponus
On Aristotle's Posterior Analytics, ed. M. Wallies, CAG XIII 3, 1909.

Plato
Laws
Theaetetus
Timaeus

Pliny the Elder
Natural History

Pliny the Younger
Letters

Plotinus
Enneads

Porphyry
Life of Plotinus

Plutarch
Platonic Questions

Rufus
Synopsis on the Pulse, ed. C. Daremberg and C.-E. Ruelle, *Oeuvres de Rufus d'Ephèse*, Paris: Imprimerie Nationale, 1879.

Seneca
Apocolyntosis
The Brevity of Life
Moral Letters
Tranquility of Mind

Sextus Empiricus
Against the Mathematicians

Simplicius
On Aristotle's On the Heavens, ed. I. L. Heiberg, CAG VII, 1894
On Aristotle's Physics, ed. H. Diels, CAG IX, 1882.

Soranus
Gynaecology, ed. J. Ilberg, CMG IV, 1927.

Stobaeus
Anthology

Suetonius
Augustus
Tiberius

Themistius
On Aristotle's Physics, ed. H. Schenkl, CAG V 2, 1900.

Secondary Literature

Armisen-Marchetti, A. (1989) *Sapientiae facies: étude sur les images de Sénèque*, Paris: Les Belles Lettres.
Armisen-Marchetti, A. (1995) 'Sénèque et l'appropriation du temps', *Latomus* 54(3): 545–67.
Arnaldi, M. and Schaldach, K. (1997) 'A Roman cylinder dial: witness to a forgotten tradition', *Journal for the History of Astronomy* 28 (2): 107–17.
Baddeley, A. (1994) 'The magical number seven: still magic after all these years', *Psychological Review* 101(2): 353–6.
Bardong, K. (1942) 'Beiträge sur Hippokrates- und Galen-Forschung', *Nachrichten von der Akademie der Wissenschaften in Göttingen, Philologisch-Historische Klasse* 7: 577–640.
Barker, A. (1978) 'Music and perception: a study in Aristoxenus', *The Journal of Hellenic Studies* 98: 9–16.
Barker, A. (1984/9) *Greek Musical Writings*, 2 vols., Cambridge: Cambridge University Press.
Barker, A. (1994) 'Ptolemy's Pythagoreans, Archytas and Plato's conception of mathematics', *Phronesis* 39: 113–35.
Barker, A. (2005) 'The journeying voice: melody and metaphysics in Aristoxenian science', *Apeiron* 38(3): 161–84.

Barton, T. S. (1994a) *Power and Knowledge: Astrology, Physiognomics, and Medicine under the Roman Empire*, Ann Arbor: University of Michigan Press.
Barton, T. S. (1994b) *Ancient Astrology*, London: Routledge.
Barton, T. S. (1995) 'Augustus and Capricorn: astrological polyvalency and imperial rhetoric', *The Journal of Roman Studies* 85: 33–41.
Beard, M. (1987) 'A complex of times: no more sheep on Romulus' birthday', *Cambridge Classical Journal* 33:1–15.
Beck, M. (2007) 'Plutarch', in de Jong and Nünlist (eds), 397–411.
Beierwaltes, W. (1967) *Plotin über Ewigkeit und Zeit: Enneade III 7*, Frankfurt am Main: Klostermann.
Ben-Dov, J. and Doering, L. (2017) (eds) *The Construction of Time in Antiquity*, Cambridge: Cambridge University Press.
Berrey, M. (2017) *Hellenistic Science at Court*, Berlin: De Gruyter.
Bettini, M. (1991) *Anthropology and Roman Culture: Kinship, Time, Images of the Soul*, Baltimore: The Johns Hopkins University Press.
Betz, H. D. (1986) *The Greek Magical Papyri in Translation, Including the Demotic Spells*, Chicago: The University of Chicago Press.
Bonnin, J. (2013) 'Horologia et memento mori: les hommes, la mort et le temps dans l'Antiquité gréco-romaine', *Latomus* 72 (2): 468–91.
Bonnin, J. (2015) *La mesure du temps dans l'Antiquité*, Paris: Les Belles Lettres.
Bonomi, S. (1984) 'Tomba Romana Del Medico a Este', *Aquileia Nostra* lv: cols. 77–107.
Borg, B. (2004a) 'Glamorous intellectuals: portraits of *pepaideumenoi* in the second and third centuries AD', in Borg (2004b), 157–78.
Borg, B. (2004b) (ed.) *Paideia: The World of the Second Sophistic*, Millennium Studies 2, Berlin: de Gruyter.
Borg, B. (2012) 'Recent approaches to the study of Roman portraits', *Perspective* 2:315–20, https://doi.org/10.4000/perspective.137 Accessed: 3.11.2021.
Boudon-Millot, V. (2009) 'Galen's *bios* and *methodos*: from ways of life to path of knowledge', in Gill et al. (eds), 175–89.
Bultrighini, I. (2018) 'Thursday (dies Iovis) in the later Roman Empire', *Papers of the British School of Rome* 86: 61–84.
Bultrighini, I. (2021a) '*Theon hemerai*: astrology, the seven-day planetary week, and the spread of astral beliefs and the cult of the seven planets in the Greco-Roman world', in I. Salvo and T. S. Scheer (eds) *Religion and Education in the Ancient Greek World*, Tübingen: Mohr Siebeck.
Bultrighini, I. (2021b) 'Calendars of the Greek East under Rome: a new look at the *Hemerologia* tables', in S. Stern (ed.) *Calendars in the Making: The Origins of Calendars from the Roman Empire to the Later Middle Ages*, 80–128, Leiden: Brill.
Carmichael, C. (1999) 'The Sabbatical/Jubilee cycle and the seven-year famine in Egypt', *Biblica* 80: 224–39.
Casperson, L. W. (2003) 'Sabbatical, Jubilee, and the Temple of Solomon', *Vetus Testamentum* 53(3): 283–96.
Cokayne, K. (2003) *Experiencing Old Age in Ancient Rome*, London: Routledge.
Coope, U. (2005) *Time for Aristotle: Physics IV.10–14*, Oxford: Oxford University Press.

Cooper, G. (2011a) *Galen, De diebus decretoriis, from Greek into Arabic: A Critical Edition, with Translation and Commentary, of Hunayn ibn Ishāq, Kitāb ayyām al-buhrān*, Farnham, Surrey: Ashgate.
Cooper, G. (2011b) 'Galen and astrology: a mésalliance?' *Early Science and Medicine* 16: 120–46.
Cooper, G. (2013) 'Approaches to the critical days in late medieval and Renaissance thinkers', *Early Science and Medicine* 18(6): 536–65.
Corbier, P. and Gascou, J. (1995) 'Inscriptions de Tébessa d'après les archives de P.-A. Février', *Antiquités africaines* 31: 277–323.
Craik, E. (2015) *The 'Hippocratic Corpus': Content and Context*, London: Routledge.
Csapo, E. and Miller, M. (1998) 'Democracy, empire, and art: toward a politics of time and narrative', in D. Boedeker and K. A. Raaflaub (eds) *Democracy, Empire, and the Arts in Fifth-Century Athens*, 87–125, Cambridge, MA: Harvard University Press.
Darbo-Peschanski (2000) (ed.) *Constructions du temps dans le monde grec ancien* Paris: CNRS Éditions.
Davidson, J. (2001) 'Dover, Foucault and Greek homosexuality: the truth of sex', *Past & Present* 170: 3–51.
Davidson, J. (2007) *The Greeks and Greek Love: A Radical Reappraisal of Homosexuality in Ancient Greece*, London: Weidenfeld and Nicolson.
Dean-Jones, L. A, (1994) *Women's Bodies in Ancient Greek Science*, Oxford: Clarendon Press.
Dench, E. (2017) 'Ethnicity, culture, and identity', in Richter and Johnson (eds), 99–114.
Denyer, N. C. (1981) 'The atomism of Diodorus Cronus', *Prudentia* 13: 33–45.
Denyer, N. C. (2009) 'Diodorus Cronus: modality, the Master Argument and formalization', *Humana Mente* 8: 33–46.
Desroches-Noblecourt, C. (1976) (ed.) *Ramsès le Grand: Catalogue de l'exposition du Grand Palais*. Paris: Galeries Nationales du Grand Palais.
Detel, W. (forthcoming) *Aristotle's Theory of Time: A New Reading*.
Dodds, E. R. (1965) *Pagans and Christians in an Age of Anxiety*, Cambridge: Cambridge University Press.
Dohrn-van Rossum, G. (1996) *History of the Hour: Clocks and Modern Temporal Orders*, Chicago: University of Chicago Press.
Dohrn-van Rossum, G. (2003) 'Clocks', in H. Cancik and H. Schneider (eds.) *Brill's New Pauly*, Leiden: Brill, 3: 458–64.
Dover, K. J. (1989) *Greek Homosexuality*, 2nd edition, London: Duckworth.
Ehrlich, S. (2012) ' "Horae" in Roman Funerary Inscriptions', Master's Thesis, The University of Western Ontario.
van der Eijk, P. J. (1999) (ed.) *Ancient Histories of Medicine: Essays in Medical Doxography in Classical Antiquity*, Leiden: Brill.
van der Eijk, P. J. (2009) 'Aristotle! What a thing for you to say!', in Gill, Whitmarsh and Wilkins (eds), 261–81.
van der Eijk, P. J. (2015a) 'On "Hippocratic" and "Non-Hippocratic" medical writings', in L. Dean-Jones and R. Rosen (eds) *Ancient Concepts of the Hippocratic: Papers Presented at the XIIIth International Hippocrates Colloquium*, 17–47, Leiden: Brill.
van der Eijk, P. J. (2015b) 'Galen on the assessment of bodily mixtures', in B. Holmes and K.-D. Fischer (eds) *The Frontiers of Ancient Science: Essays in Honor of Heinrich von Staden*, 675–98, Berlin: De Gruyter.

Emery, N., Markosian, N. and Sullivan, M. (2020) 'Time', *SEP* https://plato.stanford.edu/archives/win2020/entries/time/ Accessed: 3.11.2021.
Ewald, B. C. (1999) *Der Philosoph als Leitbild: Ikonographische Untersuchungen an römischen Sarkophagreliefs*, Mainz: P. von Zabern.
Eyben, E. (1972) 'Antiquity's view of puberty', *Latomus* 31, 677–97.
Falkner, T. M. (1990) 'The politics and poetics of time in Solon's "Ten Ages"', *The Classical Journal* 86(1): 1–15.
Fejfer, J. (2008) *Roman Portraits in Context*, Berlin: De Gruyter.
Flemming, R. (2000) *Medicine and the Making of Roman Women: Gender, Nature, and Authority from Celsus to Galen*, Oxford: Oxford University Press.
Flemming, R. (2007) 'Galen's imperial order of knowledge', in J. König and T. Whitmarsh (eds) *Ordering Knowledge in the Roman Empire*, 241–77, Cambridge: Cambridge University Press.
Flemming, R. (2019) 'Galen and the plague', in Petit (ed.), 219–44.
Garofalo, I. (2003) 'Noti sui giorni critici in Galeno', in N. Palmieri (ed.) *Rationnel et irrationnel dans la médecine ancienne et médiévale: aspects historiques, scientifiques et culturels*, 45–58, Saint-Étienne: Université de Saint-Étienne.
Gell, A. (1992) *The Anthropology of Time*, Oxford: Berg.
Gibbs, S. L. (1976) *Greek and Roman Sundials*, New Haven, CT: Yale University Press.
Gibson, S. (2005) *Aristoxenus of Tarentum and the Birth of Musicology*, London and New York: Routledge.
Gill, C., Whitmarsh, T. and Wilkins, J. (2009) (eds) *Galen and the World of Knowledge*, Cambridge: Cambridge University Press.
Goldhill, S. (2001) (ed.) *Being Greek under Rome: Cultural Identity, the Second Sophistic and the Development of Empire*, Cambridge: Cambridge University Press.
Good, J. (1968) 'Time: social organization', in D. L. Sills and R. K. Merton (eds) *International Encyclopedia of the Social Sciences*, New York: Macmillan, vol. 16: 30–42.
Gowers, E. (1995) 'The anatomy of Rome from Capitol to Cloaca', *The Journal of Roman Studies* 85: 23–32.
Graßhoff, G., Rinner, E., Schaldach, K., Fritsch, B. and Taub, L. (2015) *Ancient Sundials*, Online Database, TOPOI, https://doi.org/10.17171/1-1 Accessed: 3.11.2021.
Grmek, M. and Gourevitch, D. (1994) 'Aux sources de la doctrine médicale de Galien: l'enseignement de Marinus, Quintus et Numisianus', *ANRW* II.37.2, 1491–1528.
van Groningen, B. A. (1953) *In the Grip of the Past: Essay on an Aspect of Greek Thought*, Brill: Leiden.
Halperin, D. M. (1990) *One Hundred Years of Homosexuality; and Other Essays on Greek Love*, London: Routledge.
Halperin, D. M., Winkler, J. J. and Zeitlin, F. (1990) (eds) *Before Sexuality: The Construction of Erotic Experience in the Ancient Greek World*, Princeton, NJ: Princeton University Press.
Hankinson, R. J. (1994) 'Galen's concept of scientific progress', in *ANRW* II.37.2, 1775–89.
Hannah, R. (2005) *Greek and Roman Calendars: Constructions of Time in the Classical World*, Bristol: Bristol Classical Press.
Hannah, R. (2008) 'Timekeeping', in J. P. Oleson (ed.) *The Oxford Handbook of Engineering and Technology in the Classical World*, 740–58, Oxford: Oxford University Press.
Hannah, R. (2009) *Time in Antiquity*, New York and London: Routledge.

Hannah, R. (2011) 'The Horologium of Augustus as a sundial', *Journal of Roman Archaeology* 24: 87–95.
Hannah, R. (2013a) 'Clocks', *Encyclopedia of Ancient History*, London: Wiley-Blackwell.
Hannah, R. (2013b) 'Time in written spaces', in G. Sears, P. Keegan and R. Laurence (eds) *Written Space in the Latin West, 200 BC to AD 300*, 83–102, London and New York: Bloosmbury.
Hannah, R. (2020) 'The sundial and the calendar', in A. C. Bowen and F. Rochberg (eds) *Hellenistic Astronomy: The Science in Its Contexts*, edited by, Leiden: Brill, 323–39.
Harlow, M. E. and Laurence, R. (2002) *Growing Up and Growing Old in Ancient Rome: A Life Course Approach*, London: Routledge.
Harris, C. R. S (1973) *The Heart and the Vascular System in Ancient Greek Medicine: From Alcmaeon to Galen*, Oxford: Oxford University Press.
Haselberger, L. (2011) 'A debate on the Horologium of Augustus: controversy and clarifications', *Journal of Roman Archaeology* 24: 47–73.
Haselberger, L. (2014) (ed.) *The Horologium of Augustus: Debate and Context, Journal of Roman Archaeology*, Supplementary Series 99.
Heilen, S. (2018) 'Galen's computation of the medical weeks: textual emendations, interpretation history, rhetorical and mathematical examinations', *SCIAMUS* 19: 201–79.
Heilen, S. (2020) 'Short time in Greco-Roman astrology', in Miller and Symons (eds), 240–70.
Heslin, P. (2007) 'Augustus, Domitian and the so-called *horologium Augusti*', *The Journal of Roman Studies* 97: 1–20.
Heslin, P. (2019) 'The Julian Calendar and the Solar Meridian of Augustus: making Rome run on time', in M. P. Loar, S. C. Murray and S. Rebeggiani (eds) *The Cultural History of Augustan Rome*, 45–79, Cambridge: Cambridge University Press.
Hopkins, M. K. (1965) 'The age of Roman girls at marriage', *Population Studies* 18, 309–27.
Jenzen, I. A., and Glasemann, R. (1989) *Uhrzeiten: die Geschichte der Uhr und ihres Gebrauchs*, Frankfurt am Main: Historisches Museum Frankfurt.
de Jong, J. F. and Nünlist, R. (2007) (eds) *Time in Ancient Greek Literature*, Studies in Ancient Greek Narrative 2, Leiden: Brill.
Jones, A. (2016) (ed.) *Time and Cosmos in Greco-Roman Antiquity*, Princeton, NJ and New York: Princeton University Press and Institute for the Study of the Ancient World at New York University.
Jones, A. (2020) 'Greco-Roman sundials: precision and displacement', in Miller and Symons (eds), 125–57.
Ker, J. (2009) 'Drinking from the water-clock: time and speech in imperial Rome', *Arethusa* 42: 279–302.
Ker, J. (2020) 'Diurnal selves in ancient Rome', in Miller and Symons (eds), 184–213.
King, H. (1998) *Hippocrates' Woman: Reading the Female Body in Ancient Greece*, London: Routledge.
Kleijwegt, M. (1991) *Ancient Youth: the Ambiguity of Youth and the Absence of Adolescence in Greco-Roman Society*, Amsterdam: Gieben.
Krinis, E. (2016) 'Cyclical time in the Ismaili circle of Ikhwan al-Safa (tenth century) and in early Jewish Kabbalists circles (thirteenth and fourteenth centuries)', *Studia Islamica* 111(1): 20–108.
Kuriyama, S. (1999) *The Expressiveness of the Body and the Divergence of Greek and Chinese Medicine*, New York: Zone Books.

Landels, J. G. (1979) 'Water-clocks and time measurement in classical antiquity', *Endeavour* 3(1): 32–7.
Landes, D. S. (1983) *Revolution in Time: Clocks and the Making of the Modern World*, Cambridge, MA: Belknap Press of Harvard University Press.
Lang, J. (2012) *Mit Wissen geschmückt?: zur bildlichen Rezeption griechischer Dichter und Denker in der römischen Lebenswelt*, Wiesbaden: Reichert.
Langholf, V. (1973) ' Ὥρα—Stunde: zwei Belege aus dem Anfang des 4. Jh. v. Chr.', *Hermes* 101: 382–4.
Langholf, V. (1990) *Medical Theories in Hippocrates: Early Texts and the 'Epidemics'*, New York and Berlin: De Gruyter.
La Rocca, E. and Parisi Presicce, C. (2011) (eds) *Ritratti: le tante facce del potere*, Rome: MondoMostre.
Laurence, R. (2000) 'Metaphors, monuments and texts: the life course in Roman culture', *World Archaeology* 31:3, 442–55.
Lehoux, D. (2007) *Astronomy, Weather, and Calendars in the Ancient World: Parapegmata and Related Texts in Classical and Near-Eastern Societies*, Cambridge: Cambridge University Press.
Leith, D. (2008) 'The *diatritus* and therapy in Graeco-Roman medicine', *The Classical Quarterly* 58.2, 581–600.
Leith, D. (2021) 'Asclepiades of Bithynia as Hippocratic commentator', in P. Pormann (ed.) *Hippocrates East and West: Commentaries in the Greek, Latin, Syriac and Arabic Traditions*, 114–46, Leiden: Brill.
Lewis, M. (2000) 'Theoretical hydraulics, automata, and water clocks', in Ö. Wikander (ed.) *Handbook of Ancient Water Technology*, 343–69, Leiden: Brill.
Lewis, O. (2016) 'The practical application of ancient pulse-lore and its influence on the doctor–patient interaction', in Petridou and Thumiger (eds), 345–64.
Lewis, O. (2022) 'Galen against Archigenes on the pulse and what it teaches us about Galen's method of *diairesis*', in R. J. Hankinson and M. Havrda (eds) *Galen's Epistemology: Experience, Reason, and Method in Ancient Medicine*, 190–217, Cambridge: Cambridge University Press.
Lewis, O. (forthcoming) 'The pulse', in P. N. Singer, R. Rosen and J. Laskaris (eds) *The Oxford Handbook of Galen*, Oxford: Oxford University Press.
von Lieven, A. and Schomberg, A. (2020) 'The ancient Egyptian water clock between religious significance and scientific functionality', in Miller and Symons (eds), 52–89.
Litchfield, M. (1988) 'Aristoxenus and empiricism: a reevaluation based on his theories', *Journal of Music Theory* 32(1): 51–73.
Lloyd, G. E. R. (1979) *Magic, Reason and Experience: Studies in the Origin and Development of Greek Science*, Cambridge: Cambridge University Press.
Lloyd, G. E. R. (1988) 'Scholarship, authority and argument in Galen's *Quod animi mores*', in P. Manuli and M. Vegetti (eds) *Le opere psicologiche di Galeno*, 11–42, Naples: Bibliopolis.
Lloyd, G. E. R. (1993) 'Galen on Hellenistics and Hippocrateans: contemporary battles and past authorities', in J. Kollesch and D. Nickel (eds) *Galen und das hellenistische Erbe*, 125–43, Franz Steiner Verlag, repr. in id. (1993) *Methods and Problems in Greek Science*, 398–416, Cambridge: Cambridge University Press.

Longhi, V. (2020) *Krisis ou la décision génératrice: épopée, médecine Hippocratique, Platon*, Villeneuve d'Ascq: Presses Universitaires du Septentrion.
Loraux, N. (1986) *The Invention of Athens: The Funeral Oration in the Classical City*, trans. A. Sheridan, Cambridge, MA: Harvard University Press.
Luciani, F. (2009) 'Ultimi minuti di vita: le suddivisioni dell' hora nelle epigrafi funerarie latine', in F. Luciani, C. Maratini and A. Zaccaria Ruggiu (eds.) *Temporalia: itinerari nel tempo e sul tempo*, 121–44, Padua: Sargon.
McTaggart, J. M. E. (1908) 'The unreality of time', *Mind* 18: 457–84.
McTaggart, J. M. E. (1927) *The Nature of Existence*, Cambridge: Cambridge University Press.
Marquardt, J., Müller, I. and Helmreich, G. (1884) *Galeni Pergameni Scripta Minora*, vol. I, Leipzig: Teubner.
Marrou, H.-I. (1938) *Mousikos anēr: étude sur les scènes de la vie intellectuelle figurant sur les monuments funéraires romains*, Grenoble: Didier & Richard.
Mattern, S. M. (2008) *Galen and the Rhetoric of Healing*, Baltimore: The Johns Hopkins University Press.
Mattern, S. M. (2017) 'Galen', in Richter and Johnson (eds), 371–88.
Miller, G. A. (1956) 'The magical number seven, plus or minus two: some limits on our capacity for processing information', *The Psychological Review* 63(2): 81–97.
Miller, K. J. (2018) 'From critical days to critical hours: Galenic refinements of Hippocratic models', *TAPA* 148: 111–48.
Miller, K. J. (2020) 'Hourly timekeeping and the problem of irregular fevers', in Miller and Symons (eds), 271–92.
Miller, K. J. (forthcoming) *Doctors on the Clock: How Sundials and Water Clocks Changed Ancient Medicine*.
Miller, K. J. and Symons, S. L. (2020) (eds.) *Down to the Hour: Short Time in the Ancient Mediterranean*, Leiden/Boston: Brill.
Mitchell, S. (1993) 'Mach's mechanics and absolute space and time', *Studies in History and Philosophy of Science Part A* 24(4): 565–83.
Moraux, P. (1984) *Der Aristotelismus bei den Griechen von Andronikos bis Alexander von Aphrodisias, II: Der Aristotelismus im I. und II. Jh. n. Chr.*, Berlin and New York: De Gruyter.
Most, G. W. (1997) 'Hesiod's myth of the five (or three or four) races', *Proceedings of the Cambridge Philological Society* 43: 104–27.
Mouroutsou, G. (2020) 'The plasticity of the present moment in Marcus Aurelius' *Meditations*', *Ancient Philosophy* 40(2).
Newton-Smith, W. H. (1980) *The Structure of Time*, London: Routledge.
Nodelman, S. (1993) 'How to read a Roman portrait', in E. D'Ambra (ed.) *Roman Art in Context: An Anthology*, 10–26, Englewood Cliffs, NJ: Prentice Hall.
Nordberg, H. (1963) *Biometrical Notes: The Information on Ancient Christian Inscriptions from Rome Concerning the Duration of Life and the Dates of Birth and Death*, Acta Instituti Romani Finlandiae, II.2, Helsinki: The University Press.
Nutton, V. (1983) 'The seeds of disease: an explanation of contagion and infection from the Greeks to the Renaissance', *Medical History* 27: 1–34.
Nutton, V. (2013) *Ancient Medicine*, 2nd edition, London: Routledge.
Parkin, T. (1999) 'Ageing in antiquity: status and participation', in P. Johnson and P. Thane (eds) *Old Age from Antiquity to Post-Modernity*, 19–42, London: Routledge.

Pearson, L. (1990) *Aristoxenus: Elementa Rhythmica*, Oxford: Clarendon Press.
Pennuto, C. (2008) 'The debate on critical days in Renaissance Italy', in C. Burnett and R. Yoeli-Tlalim (eds) *Astro-Medicine: Astrology and Medicine, East and West*, 75–98, Florence: Sismel.
Petit, C. (2019) (ed.) *Galen's Treatise Περὶ ἀλυπίας (De indolentia) in Context: A Tale of Resilience*, Leiden: Brill.
Petridou, G. and Thumiger, C. (2016) (eds) *Homo Patiens: Approaches to the Patient in the Ancient World*, Leiden: Brill.
Pietrobelli, A. (2013) 'Galien agnostique: un texte caviardé par la tradition', *Revue des Études Grecques* 126: 103–35.
Pines, S. (1955) 'A tenth century philosophical correspondence', *Proceedings of the American Academy for Jewish Research* 24: 103–36.
Prosser, S. (2016) *Experiencing Time*, Oxford: Oxford University Press.
Rehak, P. (2006) *Imperium and Cosmos: Augustus and the Northern Campus Martius*, ed. J. G. Younger, Madison, WI: University of Wisconsin Press.
Remijsen, S. (2007) 'The postal service and the hour as a unit of time in antiquity', *Historia: Zeitschrift Für Alte Geschichte* 56(2): 127–40.
Richter, D. S. and Johnson, W. A. (2017) (eds) *The Oxford Handbook of the Second Sophistic*, Oxford: Oxford University Press.
Riggsby, A. M. (2009) 'For whom the clock drips', *Arethusa* 42.3, 271–8.
Romilly, J. de (1968) *Time in Greek Tragedy*, Ithaca, NY: Cornell University Press.
Roscher, W. H. (1906) 'Die Hebdomadenlehre der griechischen Philosophen und Ärzte', *Abhandlungen der sächsischen Gesellschaft* 24.6.
Rosen, R. (2004) (ed.) *Time and Temporality in the Ancient World*, Philadephia, PA: University of Pennsylvania Museum of Archaeology and Anthropology.
Rosen, R. (2010) 'Galen, satire and the compulsion to instruct', in H. J. F. Horstmanshoff and C. van Tilburg (eds) *Hippocrates and Medical Education*, 325–42, Leiden: Brill.
Rossiter, J. J. and Suksi, A. (eds) (2003) *The Seasons: Greek and Roman Perspectives*, *Mouseion* (special issue) 47.3.
Rüpke, J. (1995) *Kalender und Öffentlichkeit: Die Geschichte der Repräsentation und religiösen Qualifikation von Zeit in Rom*, Berlin: De Gruyter.
Rüpke, J. (2011) *The Roman Calendar from Numa to Constantine: Time, History, and the Fasti*, Chichester: Wiley-Blackwell.
Salas, L. (2021) *Cutting Words: Polemical Dimensions of Galen's Anatomical Experiments*, Leiden: Brill.
Salas, L. (forthcoming) 'Anatomy and physiology', in P. N. Singer, R. Rosen and J. Laskaris (eds) *The Oxford Handbook of Galen*, Oxford: Oxford University Press.
Samuel, A. E. (1972) *Greek and Roman Chronology: Calendars and Years in Classical Antiquity*, Munich: Beck.
Schadewalt, W. (1960) 'Lebenszeit und Greisenalter im frühen Griechentum', *Hellas und Hesperien*: 41–59.
Schaldach, K. (2001) *Römische Sonnenuhren: eine Einführung in die antike Gnomonik*, 3rd edn., Frankfurt-am-Rhein: Harri Deutsch.
Scheidel, W. (2001) 'Roman age structure: evidence and models', *The Journal of Roman Studies* 91: 1–26.

Schöne, H. 1933. 'Galenos' Schrift über die Siebenmonatskinder', *Quellen und Studien zur Geschichte der Naturwissenschaften und Medizin* 3 (4): 127–30.

Schütz, M. (1990) 'Zur Sonnenuhr des Augustus auf dem Marsfeld', *Gymnasium* 97, 432–57.

Sedley, D. (1977) 'Diodorus Cronus and Hellenistic philosophy', *Proceedings of the Cambridge Philological Society* 203, n.s. 23: 74–120.

Sedley, D. (2009) 'Diodorus Cronus', *SEP*, https://plato.stanford.edu/archives/win2018/entries/diodorus-cronus/ Accessed: 3.11.2021.

Sherwood, A. N., Nikolic, M., Humphrey, J. W. and Oleson, J. P. (2020) *Greek and Roman Technology: A Sourcebook of Translated Greek and Roman Texts*, 2nd edition, London: Routledge.

Shoemaker, S. (1969) 'Time without change', *The Journal of Philosophy* 19: 363–81.

Singer, P. N. (1996) 'Notes on Galen's Hippocrates', in M. Vegetti and S. Gastaldi (eds) *Studi di storia di medicina antica e medievale in memoria di Paola Manuli*, 66–76, Florence: La nuova Italia.

Singer, P. N. (1997) *Galen: Selected Works*, translated with an introduction and notes, Oxford: Oxford University Press.

Singer, P. N. (2013) (ed.) *Galen: Psychological Writings*, translated with introductions and notes by V. Nutton, D. Davies and P. N. Singer, with the collaboration of P. Tassinari, Cambridge: Cambridge University Press.

Singer, P. N. (2014) 'Galen and the philosophers: philosophical engagement, shadowy contemporaries, Aristotelian transformations', in P. Adamson, R. Hansberger and J. Wilberding (eds) *Philosophical Themes in Galen*, 7–38, London: Institute of Classical Studies.

Singer, P. N. (2019a) 'Galen and the culture of Pergamon: a view of Greek medical-intellectual life in Roman Asia', in B. Türkmen, F. Kurunaz, N. Ermiş, Y. Ekinci Danışan (eds) *II. Uluslararası Bergama Sempozyumu, 9–10 Mayıs 2013*, 131–69, Izmir.

Singer, P. N. (2019b) 'New light and old texts: Galen on his own books', in C. Petit (ed.) *Galen's Treatise Περὶ ἀλυπίας (De Indolentia) in Context: A Tale of Resilience*, 91–131, Leiden: Brill.

Singer, P. N. (2021) 'Beyond and behind the commentary: Galen on Hippocrates on elements', in P. Pormann (ed.) *Hippocrates East and West: Commentaries in the Greek, Latin, Syriac and Arabic Traditions*, 114–46, Leiden: Brill.

Singer, P. N. (2022) 'The relationship between perceptual experience and *logos*: Galen's clinical perspective', in R. J. Hankinson and M. Havrda (eds) *Galen's Epistemology: Experience, Reason, and Method in Ancient Medicine*, 156–89, Cambridge: Cambridge University Press.

Singer, P. N. (forthcoming) *Galen: Writings on Health*, translated with introduction and notes, Cambridge: Cambridge University Press.

Singer, P. N. and van der Eijk, P. J. (2018) *Galen: Works on Human Nature, vol. I: Mixtures (De temperamentis)*, translated with introduction and notes, Cambridge: Cambridge University Press.

Sipiora, P. and Baumlin, J. S. (2002) (eds) *Rhetoric and Kairos: Essays in History, Theory, and Praxis*, Albany, NY: State University of New York Press.

Siraisi, N. (1975) 'The music of pulse in the writings of Italian academic physicians (fourteenth and fifteenth centuries)', *Speculum* 50(4): 689–710.

Smith, A. (1996) 'Eternity and time', in L. Gerson (ed.) *The Cambridge Companion to Plotinus*, 196–216, Cambridge: Cambridge University Press.

Smith, W. D. (1979) *The Hippocratic Tradition*, Ithaca, NY: Cornell University Press.
Smith, W. D. (1981) 'Implicit fever theory in *Epidemics* 5 and 7', in W. F. Bynum and V. Nutton (eds) *Theories of Fever from Antiquity to the Enlightenment*, 1–18, London: Wellcome Institute for the History of Medicine, http://journals.cambridge.org/article_S0025727300070034. Accessed: 3.11.2021.
Sorabji, R. (1983) *Time, Creation and the Continuum: Theories in Antiquity and the Early Middle Ages*, London: Duckworth.
von Staden, H. (1989) *Herophilus: The Art of Medicine in Early Alexandria*, Cambridge: Cambridge University Press.
von Staden, H. (1991) 'Galen as historian', in J. A. López Férez (ed.) *Galeno: Obra, Pensamiento e Influencia*, 205–22, Madrid: Universidád Nacional de Educación a Distancia.
von Staden, H. (1992) 'The discovery of the body: human dissection and its cultural contexts in ancient Greece', *The Yale Journal of Biology and Medicine* 65: 223–41.
von Staden, H. (1997) 'Galen and the Second Sophistic', in R. Sorabji (ed.) *Aristotle and After*, 33–54, London: Institute of Classical Studies.
von Staden, H. (2004) 'Galen's Alexandria', in W. V. Harris and G. Ruffini (eds) *Ancient Alexandria between Egypt and Greece*, 179–215, Leiden: Brill.
von Staden, H. (2006) 'Interpreting "Hippokrates" in the 3rd and 2nd centuries BC', in C. W. Müller et al. (eds) *Ärzte und ihre Interpreten*, 15–47, Berlin: De Gruyter.
von Staden, H. (2009) 'Staging the past, staging oneself: Galen on Hellenistic exegetical traditions', in Gill et al. (eds), 132–56.
Steele, J. M. (2016) (ed.) *The Circulation of Astronomical Knowledge in the Ancient World*, Leiden: Brill.
Stern, S. (2012) *Calendars in Antiquity: Empires, States, and Societies*, Oxford: Oxford University Press.
Swain, S. (1996) *Hellenism and Empire: Language, Classicism and Power in the Greek World AD 50–250*, Oxford: Clarendon Press.
Talbert, R. J. A. (2017) *Roman Portable Sundials: the Empire in Your Hand*, Oxford: Oxford University Press.
Talbert, R. J. A. (2020) 'Roman concern to know the hour in broader historical context', in A. Belousov and C. J. Ilyushechkina (eds.) *Homo Omnium Horarum: Symbolae Ad Anniversarium Septuagesimum Professoris Alexandri Podosinov Dedicatae*, 534–55, Moscow: Academia Pozharskiana.
Tempest-Walters, K. (2020) 'A Translation of and Commentary on Plotinus' *Ennead* III.7', Ph.D Dissertation, Royal Holloway, University of London.
Thompson, E. P. (1967) 'Time, work-discipline, and industrial capitalism', *Past & Present* 38: 56–97.
Totelin, L. (2009) *Hippocratic Recipes: Oral and Written Transmission of Knowledge in Fifth- and Fourth-Century Greece*, Leiden: Brill.
Totelin, L. (2021) 'A woman in flux: fluidity in Hippocratic gynaecology', in C. Thumiger (ed.) *Holism in Ancient Medicine and its Reception*, 220–36, Leiden: Brill.
Trédé-Boulmer, M. (2015) *Kairos, L'à-propos et l'occasion: Le mot et la notion d'Homère à la fin du IVe siècle avant J.-C.*, revised edition, Paris: Les Belles Lettres.
Turetzky, P. (1998) *Time*, London: Routledge.
Turner, A. (1990 *Time*, The Hague: Tijd voor Tijd Foundation.

Vegetti, M. (1999a) 'Tradition and truth: forms of philosophical–scientific historiography in Galen's *De placitis*', in van der Eijk (ed.), 333–57.
Vegetti, M. (1999b) 'Historiographical strategies in Galen's physiology (*De usu partium, De naturalibus facultatibus*)', in van der Eijk (ed.), 383–95.
Vegetti, M. (2001) 'Il confronto degli antichi e dei moderni in Galeno', in G. Cajani and D. Lanza (eds) *L'antico degli antichi*, 87–100, Palermo: Palumbo.
Vegetti, M. (2013) *Galeno: Nuovi scritti autobiografici: introduzione traduzione e commento*, Rome: Carocci Editore.
Wallace-Hadrill, A. (1987) 'Time for Augustus: Ovid, Augustus and the *Fasti*', in M. Whitby and P. Hardie (eds) *Homo viator: Classical Essays for John Bramble*, 221–30, Bristol: Bristol Classical Press.
Walters, J. (1997) 'Invading the Roman body: manliness and impenetrability in Roman thought', in J. P. Hallett, J. P. and M. B. Skinner (eds) *Roman Sexualities*, 29–46, Princeton, NJ: Princeton University Press.
West, M. L. (1971) 'The cosmology of "Hippocrates", *De hebdomadibus*', *The Classical Quarterly* 21(2): 365–88.
West, M. L. (1992) *Ancient Greek Music*, Oxford: Clarendon Press.
Whitmarsh, T. J. G. (2001) *Greek Literature and Roman Identities: The Politics of Imitation*, Oxford: Oxford University Press.
Whitmarsh, T. J. G. (2007) 'Philostratus', in de Jong and Nünlist (eds), 413–30.
Wiedemann, T. (1989) *Adults and Children in the Roman Empire*, London: Routledge.
Winkler, J. J. (1990) *The Constraints of Desire: The Anthropology of Sex and Gender in Ancient Greece*, London: Routledge.
Winter, E. (2013) *Zeitzeichen: zur Entwicklung und Verwendung antiker Zeitmesser*, 2 vols., Berlin: De Gruyter.
Wolkenhauer, A. (2011) *Sonne und Mond, Kalender und Uhr: Studien zur Darstellung und poetischen Reflexion der Zeitordnung in der römischen Literatur*, Untersuchungen zur antiken Literatur und Geschichte, Berlin: De Gruyter.
Wolkenhauer, A. (2020) 'Time, punctuality, and chronotopes: concepts and attitudes concerning short time in ancient Rome', in Miller and Symons (eds), 214–38.
Zanker, P. (1988) *The Power of Images in the Age of Augustus*, trans. A. Shapiro, Ann Arbor: University of Michigan Press.

Index of names

d'Abano, Pietro 121
Aeneas Tacticus 13, 165
Aëtius of Amida 64, 166
Agathinus 87
Ammonius 99
Anaxagoras 17
Anaximander 6
Annia Faustina 29
Antoninus Pius (emperor) 2
Antyllus 64, 81
Apollo 9, 77
Archigenes 83, 87 f., 141
Ariston 86, 88
Aristotle 14, 36 f., 41–44, 47 f., 75 f., 79, 86, 125–135, 152, 156, 166, 169
– *Physics* 125–127, 129–131, 133, 166, 169
– *Politics* 41, 43 f., 166
– *Rhetoric* 36 f., 44, 166
Aristoxenus of Tarentum 128, 144, 156–159, 164, 166
– *Elements of Harmonics* 159, 166
– *Elements of Rhythm* 156, 166
Asclepiades of Bithynia 75, 83, 87 f., 92
– Asclepiadean 75
Asclepius 77 f., 95, 99
Asinius Pollio 32
Athenaeus of Attalia 64, 166
Athenaeus of Naucratis 7, 14 f., 83, 87 f.
Augustus (emperor) 1, 5, 32, 38, 65, 67, 169
Aulus Gellius 27, 167

Bodier, Thomas 121

Caelius Aurelianus 110
Cardano, Girolamo 121
Chrysippus 75, 79, 86
Cicero 17, 24, 26, 32, 85, 166
Commodus (emperor) 29, 90
Ctesibius 15 f.

Damascius 152, 166
Demosthenes 14, 166

Dieuches 83, 87
Dio Cassius 38 f., 166
Diocles of Carystus 75, 83, 87 f.
Diodorus Cronus 127
Diogenes Laertius 6, 41, 166
Dodds, Eric Robertson 90

Empedocles of Acragas 43, 77 f.
Epictetus 70, 166
Erasistratus of Ceos 73, 75, 83, 87 f., 92, 95
Eudemus 60, 87 f.
Euripides 38, 167
Euryphon 86, 88

Favorinus of Arles 87
Fracastoro, Girolamo 121

Galen 8 f., 18–24, 26, 28–33, 36 f., 41, 43 f., 46–52, 58–62, 64, 71–100, 106–123, 127–162, 164–167
– *Affections and Errors of the Soul* 18, 94, 167
– *An Exhortation to Study the Arts* 167
– *Anatomical Procedures* 79, 85, 94, 167
– *Bloodletting against Erasistratus* 95, 167
– *Commentary on Hippocrates' Aphorisms* 60, 86, 88, 167
– *Commentary on Hippocrates'; Epidemics* 46, 49, 52, 61, 85, 167
– *Commentary on Hippocrates' The Nature of the Human Being* 49, 85, 167
– *Crises* 103, 107, 116 f., 167
– *Critical Days* 47, 106 f., 112, 118 f., 121, 167
– *Health* 30 f., 33, 47–51, 60, 81, 137, 167
– *Mixtures* 47, 58, 83, 145 f., 167
– *My Own Books* 61, 92–95, 167
– *Periods* 107 f., 112–115, 167
– *Prognosis* 28 f., 60 f., 90, 94, 107 f., 110 f., 167
– *Synopsis on the Pulse* 154, 167, 169

– *The Best Doctor is Also a Philosopher* 84, 89 f.
– *The Discernment of the Pulse* 140–143, 146 f., 149–151, 153, 155, 167
– *The Distinct Types of Fever* 59, 107, 112 f., 167
– *The Distinct Types of Pulse* 136, 138, 144, 156, 167
– *The Doctrines of Hippocrates and Plato* 60, 75, 77, 79, 85, 167
– *The Order of My Own Books* 93, 97, 167
– *The Pulse for Beginners* 60, 141, 167
– *The Shaping of the Embryo* 96, 167
– *The Soul's Dependence on the Body* 44, 75, 96, 167
– *The Therapeutic Method* 49, 78, 83, 87, 89, 107, 111 f., 167
– *The Therapeutic Method to Glaucon* 49, 107, 167
Gibbon, Edward 90
Gordian (emperor) 99

Herodotus (historian) 6 f., 167
Herodotus (medical author) 81
Herophilus of Chalcedon 27 f., 73, 87 f., 123, 136, 141, 152–158, 160–162, 164
Hesiod 37, 52, 72, 75, 77 f., 167
'Hippocrates'
– historical figure and Galen's attitude to 46, 58, 60, 73–78, 80–84, 86–88, 108, 113, 118
– *Affections* 18 f., 21, 23, 89, 94, 104, 167
– *Airs, Waters, Places* 56, 168
– *Aphorisms* 45, 47, 56–58, 60, 87 f., 102, 106, 167 f.
– *Diseases* 104, 168
– *Diseases of Girls* 45, 168
– *Epidemics* 7, 46, 49, 52, 55 f., 61, 85, 107, 113, 167 f.
– *Hebdomads* 36, 41 f., 46, 52, 168
– *Internal Affections* 7, 168
– *Regimen* 29, 35 f., 44, 47, 52 f., 57, 59, 168
– *Regimen in Acute Diseases* 86, 104, 168
– *Regimen in Health* 57, 59, 168
– *The Nature of the Human Being* 36, 56–59, 108, 167 f.

Hippocratic corpus 7 f., 36, 38, 73, 104, 106
Homer 37 f., 52, 82, 168
Horace 37, 168

Ibn Abī Saʿīd 132

Julius Caesar 5

Lepidus 5

Machon 7
Magni, Antonio 121
Mainardi, Giovanni 121
Marcellinus 28, 160, 168
Marcus Aurelius (emperor) 31 f., 70, 90, 96, 111, 168
Marinus (medical author) 78, 84 f., 87 f.
Martial 25 f.
Methodist (school of medicine) 8, 29, 75, 78, 80 f., 87 f., 110–112
Mirandola, Pico della 121
Mnesitheus 83, 87

Oresme, Nicolas 121
Ovid 36, 72, 168

Parmenides 125, 152
Pausanias 77, 104
Peitholaus 29
Pericles 17, 36
Pertinax (emperor) 93
Petronius 3, 69, 168
Pherecydes 86, 88
Philistion 77 f., 86, 88
Philoponus, John 156, 168
Philostratus 98
Philotimus 87 f.
Plato 7, 14 f., 43 f., 47, 74–76, 81 f., 86, 96, 124–126, 132, 135, 152, 166, 168
– *Laws* 7, 44, 168
– *Theaetetus* 14, 168
– *Timaeus* 44, 124, 152, 166, 168
Plautus 27
Pleistonicus 87
Pliny (the Elder) 2, 6, 13, 17, 25, 27, 30, 168

Pliny (the Younger) 3, 17, 21, 31, 37, 168
Plotinus 98–101, 124f., 168
Plutarch of Chaeronea 98, 125, 168
Polybus 86, 88
Porphyry 74, 98–100, 168
– *Life of Plotinus* 98–101, 168
Posidonius 86
Praxagoras of Cos 75, 87f., 136
Ptolemy 20, 119, 121
Pythagoras 41

Quintus (medical author) 84, 87f., 90

Rufus of Ephesus 87, 154, 168f.

Sabinus (medical author) 87

Seneca (the Younger) 17, 27, 32, 37, 69–71, 169
Sextus Empiricus 127, 169
Simplicius 22, 125, 128, 130–132, 169
Soranus of Ephesus 48, 110, 169
Spurinna 26, 30
Stobaeus 64, 169
Suetonius 32, 38, 169

Themistius 128–134, 169
Theophrastus 75, 86
Thessalus (Methodist) 77f., 80f.
Tiberius (emperor) 32, 38, 169

Vitruvius 15f., 20

General index

accuracy   4, 6f., 15, 17f., 20f., 24, 40, 48, 61, 67f., 86, 105, 120, 138, 142, 145, 148, 153f., 157f., 160, 164
adulescens: see youth
age
– golden   72, 75, 77f., 89
– (= stage of life)   29f., 35–44, 46–51, 56f., 60, 63–66, 72f., 75, 77–79, 88–90, 94–96, 99f., 100, 103, 143, 145f., 153f., 158, 160
– old   29f., 37–47, 49–51, 60, 64f., 72, 74, 77, 79, 81, 83, 88, 154f.
– see also child; *hēbē*; post-prime; prime; puberty; transitional; youth
aiōn: see eternity
Alexandria   31, 72f., 85, 95
analēmma   20
ancient (authors, etc.)   1–4, 8, 10–12, 19–21, 24, 28, 31f., 36–42, 46f., 52f., 59, 66, 68, 72–76, 78–85, 87, 91, 93f., 96, 98f., 102–104, 106–110, 117f., 120, 122f., 125, 135, 137, 139–141, 143, 146, 153, 157, 159, 161f., 164
– see also *palaios*
architect   20, 82
architecture   15, 20
astrology, astrological   35, 41, 67, 69, 102, 117–119, 121
astronomy, astronomer, astronomical   10, 35, 77, 82, 118, 121, 125; see also sphere, celestial
atomic, atomist, atomistic   124, 127f., 148, 152, 158, 162

Babylonian   6
bath, bathing   25f., 28–32
biography   66f., 72, 91, 94, 96, 98–100

calendar   4–6, 33, 55, 69
child, childhood   37–39, 41, 44, 47, 49, 65, 67, 104, 153f.
clepsydra: see water-clock
Cnidus   77–78

Cos   77f.
crisis (of disease): *see krisis*
cycle   33, 35–38, 41, 51, 55f., 60f., 63, 65f., 102, 106, 114, 118–122

day   1f., 4–9, 13, 18f., 21–23, 25–33, 37, 53, 55f., 58, 64, 67–70, 72, 76–78, 90, 92, 102, 106–108, 110–122, 132, 137, 142, 148, 161, 167
– critical   47, 92, 102, 106f., 112, 117–119; see also krisis
diastolē: see pulse, expansion of
diatritus   110–112
disease: see diatritus; fever; mixture; periodic; plague

education   9, 20, 43, 46–48, 72f., 77, 80, 94, 110
Egypt   6, 14
– Egyptian   14f.
ephebate   39
ephēbos: see youth
episode (of fever)   28, 103, 106, 108, 112f., 120
equinox   13, 22, 31, 53f., 56
era, golden; *see* age
eternity   2, 9, 70, 124f.
exercise   1, 25–27, 29–32, 35, 48, 57, 59; see also regime, daily

festivals, festive time   5, 33f.
fever   28f., 45, 47, 49, 56, 58–60, 62, 102f., 106–108, 110f., 113–116, 118, 120, 122, 160
– continuous   58f., 108, 111, 116, 124, 127, 129, 150–152, 158, 162
– quartan   47, 58–60, 108, 113–116, 118
– quotidian   60, 108, 113–116
– tertian   58, 60, 108, 113–116, 118
– see also episode; *krisis*; periodic; periodicity; recurrence

fluid (humoral, of body) ; *see also* mixture 30, 36, 40 f., 47, 51, 59 f., 62 f., 75, 85, 108
future   69–71, 94, 98, 107, 124

gnomon   6, 10, 18–20, 151
gymnasium   4, 24 f., 29, 32

hebdomad   36, 41–44, 46 f., 49, 52, 94, 168
hēbē   43, 45, 48
hōra: see hour; season
horologium   1–3, 5 f.
hour   1–4, 6–13, 15, 17, 20–33, 67–70, 102, 110–116, 120 f., 140
– equinoctial   1, 9, 31 f.
– seasonal   1, 4, 6 f., 9, 13, 23, 32 f., 52, 58–61, 63

instant, ceasing   70, 127, 152

kairos   102–106, 111 f.
krisis   102–106, 111

lawcourt   1 f., 4, 13 f., 16 f., 24, 26, 39 f., 103, 106
legal: *see* lawcourt
leisure   1, 4, 26, 31 f.

meirakion: see youth
mental   33, 50, 69–71, 133–135, 145, 147–149, 151, 157, 164
Mesopotamia   6
mixture (of body or fluids)   43, 49, 58, 119, 128, 145
– badly-mixed   119
– well-mixed   30, 119
modern   3, 9, 14, 19, 32, 41, 65, 68 f., 76, 78, 82–84, 88 f., 93, 96 f., 101, 106, 108, 113, 117, 121, 135–137, 141, 147 f., 161, 165
– early   1, 4, 6 f., 15, 17, 36, 48, 52, 65, 79, 92, 94, 99 f., 104–106, 117, 121, 126, 135, 143
– *see also neōteros, neōteroi*
moment
– transitional   37–39

– *see also* instant; present
motion   6, 32, 52–54, 88, 118, 123–127, 129–136, 138, 140–142, 145–147, 149–152, 155–158, 160, 162
music   77, 128, 143 f., 148, 156 f.
– theory   8, 41, 43, 46, 75 f., 79, 82 f., 88, 102, 117–119, 121, 127 f., 136, 141, 146, 152–154, 156, 158–160, 162

neaniskos: see youth
Neoplatonist   125
neōteros, neōteroi   65, 74 f., 77, 79–81, 83–89, 97, 104, 112, 118, 120, 135, 147, 165
night   4, 6, 8, 13, 24, 27 f., 31 f., 54, 57, 64, 113, 167

paideia: see education
palaios, palaioi (in Galen's construction of the past) 74 f., 77, 79, 81–89, 109
parapēgma   55
past   14, 69–72, 74 f., 77, 81–83, 86, 89, 94, 97, 124, 127, 152
peira   102, 106, 111
Pergamum   9, 24, 61
periodic (disease, illness, fever)   7, 28, 61, 106–108, 113, 117 f., 122
periodicity   29, 35, 109 f., 118, 120, 122; *see also* recurrence
periodization   75, 83, 85 f., 88, 97
philosopher   6, 17 f., 37, 69, 76, 79, 82 f., 86, 94, 152, 166
philosophy   9, 73, 76, 90, 92, 94, 99, 135
plague   51, 61, 96–98
Pompeii   9, 18
post-prime   46, 49 f., 60, 103, 154
precision: *see* accuracy
present (time or moment)   69–72, 74, 77–79, 82, 90, 97, 124, 127, 152, 160, 164
prime (as stage of life) 37, 41, 43 f., 46–50, 56, 60, 100, 103, 154
puberty   38, 40, 43–45, 48
pulse   27–29, 60–62, 83, 92, 107, 112, 123, 136–147, 149 f., 152–155, 158–163, 168
– contraction of   136–138, 141–143, 149, 153–156
– expansion of   136–138, 141–143, 147, 149, 152–156

quantification   40, 123, 159, 161f., 164

ratio   123, 136f., 140, 142, 148, 152–157, 162
recent, more (authors or doctors, in Galen's view): *see neōteros*
recurrence 7, 28, 35, 61, 108–110, 113, 116, 118, 120; *see also* periodicity
regime, daily   7, 26, 28–33, 48, 51, 95, 111; *see also* exercise
rhythm   123, 127f., 137, 148, 152–155, 157–159, 162, 164
Rome   1–5, 10, 13, 31, 61, 67, 81, 85, 87f., 90, 92, 95f., 99
– Ara Pacis   1, 3
– Campus Martius   1–3, 5
– forum   1f., 17, 29f., 96

season   4, 6f., 23, 30, 34–36, 41, 46, 51–53, 55–61, 63f., 102
'Second Sophistic'   72, 74
solstice   4, 13, 22, 31, 58

soul   44, 48, 50, 66, 71, 75f., 96, 124f., 152
speed   14f., 50, 53f., 106, 123, 125, 128, 136, 138–143, 145–148, 150f., 153, 157–162, 164
sphere, celestial   9f., 52–54, 125
– two-sphere model of cosmos   52–54, 125
Stoic   69–71, 75, 79, 87, 92, 126
sundial   1–6, 8–13, 17–24, 27, 120, 151
systolē: see pulse, contraction of

transitional (moment, phase, stage)   38f., 45, 49, 58

water-clock   1–4, 8, 13–17, 21–24, 27, 69, 159–161
woman, women   36, 38, 163

youth   37–39, 41–44, 46–50, 64f., 84, 96, 104f., 111, 144, 154

zodiac   4f., 15, 53f., 118

www.ingramcontent.com/pod-product-compliance
Lightning Source LLC
Chambersburg PA
CBHW061348300426
44116CB00011B/2040